Action learning in hospitals
Diagnosis and therapy

Other titles from McGRAW-HILL Book Company (UK) Limited

Cortazzi and Roote: Illuminative Incident Analysis
Lynch: The People Power Gap
Hamblin: Evaluation and Control of Training
Adair: Action Centered Leadership

Action learning in hospitals
Diagnosis and therapy

Professor R. W. Revans

London . New York . St Louis . San Francisco . Auckland .
Düsseldorf . Johannesburg . Kuala Lumpur . Mexico.
Montreal . New Delhi . Panama . Paris . São Paulo .
Singapore . Sydney . Tokyo . Toronto

Published by McGRAW-HILL Book Company (UK) Limited
MAIDENHEAD · BERKSHIRE · ENGLAND

07 084470 4

Library of Congress Cataloging in Publication Data

Main entry under title:

Action learning in hospitals.

    Pt. 1 of this book originally published in 1964 under title: Standards of morale.
    1. Hospitals—Personnel management. 2. Hospitals—Staff—In-service training. 3. Hospitals Internal Communications Project. I. Revans, Reginald W., 1907–　II. Revans, Reginald W., 1907–　Standards for morale. 1976. [DNLM: 1. Hospitals for personnel administration. 2. Attitude of health personnel. 3. Morale. WX159 R449s]
RA971.35.A25　　658.3′7′36211　　76-6068
ISBN 0-07-084470-4

5 4 3 2 1 PPPP 79876

TEXT SET IN 11/12PT PHOTON TIMES, PRINTED BY PHOTOLITHOGRAPHY,
AND BOUND IN GREAT BRITAIN AT THE PITMAN PRESS, BATH

Foreword

I first met the chief author of this book when he joined the staff of Manchester University as Professor of Industrial Administration. His main work had been on the subject of the management of coal mines, about which I knew nothing. I found his exposition of his subject quite fascinating, partly because it was practical, but more because it was analytical and had taken full account of the human factors involved; a study based not on intuition but on reputable techniques of interviews and statistical correlations. The correlation between sickness absence and staff relations I found particularly interesting as a doctor.

When Professor Revans turned his attention towards the National Health Service I was, of course, even more interested. He found great similarities in matters such as staff morale which, in hospitals as in industry, starts at the top and goes right through every level. (You can sense it straight away when you telephone—the cold 'hold the line' followed by ten minutes' silence, contrasted with a courteous 'I'm so sorry, I'll try again to locate him'.)

Professor Revans doesn't happen to have included telephonists specifically in his research, but he is most interesting on the extent to which wastage among trainee nurses, length of stay in hospital, sickness among nurses, and other factors, correlated with the attitudes of senior and junior doctors. It all comes down to the standard of morale in a hospital, and the genius of Professor Revans's research, fully described in this book, lies in the methods used in assessing all the factors involved. To have got ten major hospitals to collaborate in the task is a considerable achievement.

If this book is as widely read as it deserves to be, it could make a major contribution to the prevention of the periodic 'industrial action' and threats of mass resignation which have been such a degrading feature of the Health Service in recent times. Cool examination of the facts, and positive collaboration between management and professions, is surely what is needed. The former dignity of the medical profession has indeed reached an interesting stage when one who learnt his skill in the study of the coal-mining industry is an appropriate investigator.

Lord Platt of Grindleford, MD, FRCP
formerly President, Royal College of Physicians

Table of Contents

Preface

This is a book about an action learning project, based on research in hospital organization first published as *Standards for Morale* in 1964. This earlier book, revised and reproduced in this volume, recommended experiments in action learning to improve hospital effectiveness. Whatever action learning may be will not necessarily become clear simply by reading what the present writers have to say about it, since the book is but a river of words. It is at most a silent memorial to the past activities of many people, and is no more what they actually did than could any current biography of Napoleon be that very man himself, marching in his resurrection on Brussels with a knapsack full of new grievances. Action learning is *both to understand and to achieve* as a result of trying out, perhaps more than once, some suggestion for reaching an objective; it is even more itself if, at the outset, the objective itself is not entirely clear: learning by doing then becomes learning what to be doing. Indeed, the achievement *is* necessarily the understanding: to know is to be able to do and the outcome is the knowledge. Action learning is thus an expression of the philosophy of pragmatism as taught by William James of Harvard and John Dewey of Columbia: that what is useful is true and that which cannot be used cannot be assumed to exist and hence cannot be true. It is thus a descendant of Franciscan experimentation and agrees with William of Ockham (*c.* 1340): 'Essences are not to be multiplied without necessity.' It is both necessary and sufficient to demonstrate that something suggested can be done; there is no need to introduce intermediate arguments to connect different parts of its doing with each other. Werner Heisenberg demonstrated the same economy in his theories of atomic behaviour in 1926.

In the words of Sophocles: 'It is doing the thing that counts. For although you may think you know it, you have no certainty until you try it.' So with this book. Its readers may feel that they now understand action learning, whereas they have merely read what others have written about it. Only if the book inspires a few to have a go at action learning themselves—as the stagey violence of television is said to unleash the private violence of those who watch—can their apprenticeship as action learners be held to have started.

Our main illustration, drawn by Janet Craig, is of action learning in a group of London hospitals. It was a complex and painful exercise, well charged with Nietzschean foreboding: that nothing new can be accepted unless it is first both ridiculed and opposed. At times, it seemed as if Janet Craig alone believed the experiment worth pursuing. And yet our goal was simplicity itself. Could their staffs learn how to make those hospitals more efficient by themselves setting about what needed to be discovered, defined, treated and changed–all in the *we-here-and-now* of daily practice? To normal persons (as those who have tried to answer this question in the real hospital world have found out, and they are a band small and select compared with those who feel it enough merely to ratiocinate about that world in order to improve it), the question seems unnecessary. For why, asks Common Sense, should any staff, whether concerned with patients, or with maintenance or supplies or records or even cooking, need to spend their own precious time in studying or changing their established work order? Is it not the task of hospital administrators to look after all that? If it is not their job, what right have administrators to be where they are? Or, even if the administration eventually admits that it can do little about such troubles, because it is, for example, too busy on planning a new hospital, could it not engage management consultants to put them right? If not, what are all the management consultants there for, anyhow? Or, should the consultants admit that the problems are outside their expert field, could not the administrators invite *real* research workers in, such as the professors from university departments of organizational behaviour or intervention science? ... What, then, can be the possible justification, in the face of all these experts, for distracting the hospital staff themselves by such extraordinary exercises as their involvement in how their work is done?

One answer to some of these questions given by the student of Sophocles, by the philosopher committed to doing things as well as to talking about them, would be that the operational problems of so complex a system as a hospital cannot be understood in any external or objective or detached sense, that is, other than by being involved in handling them: the very problems themselves take on meaning only in needing to solve them, just as medical science has evolved out of studying not the healthy but the sick. Another answer would be that, even if the detached analysis was a faithful representation of the reality, it still has to be interpreted by those who work in that reality. The concept of action learning implies not only that one learns *to solve problems only by the act of solving them*, but also that in this way alone does one learn to trace an effective solution among the many choices available. Even this is not all. Any grasp of the idea of action learning demands that one also engages in action learning as the only way of mastering what action learning may be. Such engagement is likely only long after all else has been seen to fail. Thus, until it has been more widely recognized that one solves material problems neither by simulating them in a classroom nor by making speeches about them, nor by writing books about them—'It hath not pleased God to grant his people salvation in dialectic' (Ambrose, *De Fide*, i, v, 42)—there can be no motivation among teachers to expose their traditional scholarship to the uncharitable scrutiny of daily circumstance. Thus the conventional wisdom of the National Health Service continues to have it that money alone is necessary to its salvation; the old principles of management, imposed in the old way, but smartened and stiffened here and there with a computer or a bit of PERT, disposing of a few hundred million pounds and all would again be well.

... And yet? Is it unreasonable to suggest that, in real terms, such money will never again be available and that other quests for improvement will need to be pursued? ... We remain ready to diffuse our convictions about action learning elsewhere in the social services.

No claim, however, is being made, either for exclusiveness or originality in support of action learning; others in the field of managerial development are trying it out as well (see *The Making of a Manager: A World View*, Sidney Mailick (ed.), Anchor Press/Doubleday, New York, 1972, especially chapters 4 and 8). If this particular tract on the topic has any slender merit (apart from its emphasis that a knowledge of the literature is no claim to know the subject), it is probably to be found partly in the verification of the experiment itself, partly in its references to pioneer action learning elsewhere. There is, on the one hand, little to be lost by any experiments producing the results predicted in their design, and, on the other, no overwhelming reason for condemning experiments in the social field that conform to this convention. The hospital study, since it began ten years ago, has now had time enough to exhibit its consequences, and the account of Margaret and Kenneth Ulyatt (Part Three) about its outcome is an interesting contribution to social research, for, despite the roughness of their statistical material and the robust simplicity of their methods, the results of the experiment are clearly to be seen. The five London hospitals, in which a few of the staff eventually grasped what action learning might be, showed improvements in the use of their resources significantly greater than those of comparable hospitals that either did not join the experiment or that joined but had difficulty in understanding what action learning could achieve. This work of the Ulyatts has brought forcibly home the universal need for better and more discriminating records of ward experience: there can be no substantial improvement in future programmes of patient care until we have reasonably accurate ways of describing the programmes now on offer, and reliable statistics are one of these.

Our tract closes with an essay by Nelson Coghill (Part Five) on possible developments in action learning. His thesis is that, whatever management theory or administrative science may have to offer (as, for example, the White Papers of the Department of Health and Social Security on the reorganization of the National Health Service) for our guidance through the darkening labyrinths of our new Leviathan, there will always be some place, modest enough, perhaps, for the ideas and efforts of those who carry out the subordinate tasks. We may in the past have had just a little too much regard for the advice of the literate élite, just as we may, perhaps, have had too much respect for their convenience. In an economy in which quite ordinary people, such as coalminers and shipyard workers, have discovered not only how to defy governments but also to destroy them, it may be well to find out what such people may be feeling about their work. Since actions still speak louder than words, we might identify these feelings by encouraging their natural expression in the course of the work itself, no less than through their complaints about its difficulties and their claims for its rewards. Action learning offers one opportunity. By providing the conditions in which persons can cooperate in the antecedent design and subsequent review of their own tasks, a few managements are opening to their organizations a new quest for efficiency and for morale; Mr Wedgwood Benn is boldly encouraging some workers to think about being their own bosses. Much of our present confusion about worker consultation, worker participation and worker control can be traced to one simple failure: we do not sufficiently appreciate that what concerns the workman most, what absorbs the greatest share of his life, and what he knows more about than all others in the world, is the job at which he gains his living. Nothing is more a part of him than is the very job he does. This book is very much an illustration of how such self-involvement in one's own job may be secured.

R. W. Revans
A.L.P. International
London: 1976

PART ONE

Standards for Morale

by Professor R. W. Revans

Preface to the 1976 edition

Since this work was first published in 1964, the National Health Service has been reorganized; two major changes have overtaken the nursing profession, a new hierarchy of nursing officers was created as recommended by the Salmon Report and in 1974 this hierarchy was changed yet again to fit in with the structure of the new Health Service. There are no longer for example, any matrons, deputy matrons or home sisters. Changes in the education system, too, have led to some cadet schemes being discontinued. But we have decided not to make all the consequential amendments and omissions that these changes might demand in our text; after all, it is by no means certain that the structure of the senior nursing staff will remain as it is or that cadet schemes will not once more find a firm place in the educational system. Indeed, as for cadets, all the evidence is that the development of the adolescent in Britain is not quite the piece of academic cake it was once thought to be. From what one hears of the problems of some schools, the hospital cadet scheme may be in for a major revival.

Foreword to the 1964 edition

These studies of life in hospital occupied nearly 20 persons from time to time over the course of five years. Their detailed organization in the field was due to James A. Fraser, lately lecturer in psychology in the University of Manchester; his help and his help alone made much of the survey possible. A lifetime of practical experience gave him an insight into the behaviour of ordinary people and an ease in reassuring them without which the work would have got little beyond the arid analysis of hospital statistics; he has continued to help and advise in his retirement. Much of the collection of statistics was carried out, with an astonishing blend of tact, audacity and success by William Staton, lately Director of Education to the Borough of Leyton; he was helped by Kenneth Wallis, now lecturer at Regent Street Polytechnic; Dr Vera Bruce Chambers conducted the survey of nursing cadet schemes and found herself on the General Nursing Council at the end of it; John Pantall, now tutor to students of hospital administration under Professor T. E. Chester, spent four years working with James Fraser on field work that ranged from attitude surveys to the direction of a team of analysts sampling ward activities. Dr Mahendra Srivastava from Cawnpore first made order of hospital statistics by his diligent searches into the records of thousands of nurses; Dr Noorali Nanji from Nairobi reduced the opinions of hundreds of ward sisters to a form that the Manchester computer could handle. Miss Hilary Hutty lent a hand at everything, living in nurses' homes, interviewing matrons, writing up gigantic attitude surveys, typing this report. Other members of staff who became involved included John Beresford, lately of the Operational Research group of the National Coal Board, and Jack Butterworth, head of the College work study section. The project was directed and written up by Reginald W. Revans, who alone must be responsible for its obscurities and misconceptions.

Introduction to the 1964 edition

The adjustment to change

This essay describes the work and conclusions of a small group at the Manchester College of Science and Technology (none of whom was medically qualified); we spent about four years in a number of hospitals, mainly in the North of England, observing, discussing and analysing a variety of human problems, beginning with the adjustment of the student nurse to her professional task. Our group was drawn from the Department of Industrial Administration; its members could claim previous research in the field of organization and some had had responsible experience of industrial management. The Department is generally attempting to bring the methods of operational research and of work study to the analysis of administration; as far as possible our team has used techniques of direct observation and of statistical analysis in these particular studies of hospital problems, and the essay is based exclusively upon our own research material. (This is not to suggest that there is any lack of other studies, nor that among these there is none more worthwhile than this.)

Others of the Department's hospital studies find no place in this report, although the Department has had hospital and nursing staff through its work study courses and has eventually been engaged with them upon problems of hospital transport systems, hospital committee structures, hospital stores, hospital costing systems, hospital laundries, and the organization of a hospital matron's office. It is as well to mention these practical assignments, since there is a tendency to regard university research workers in the field of social science as interested only in remote abstractions, and to judge their findings of little account in the world of unsympathetic reality. That those who made this study and wrote this report are lay amateurs makes it more necessary to stress their respect for observation; it may also help to excuse the accent in this report on statistical material. Such evidence does not, of course, impress everybody and we do not expect it to do so; we may, however, make some impact by emphasizing the first-handedness of much of our observation. When, for the first time, one's enquiries on the floor of the hospital bring one to share baked beans on toast at two o'clock on a Sunday morning with the night staff, the conversation is not likely to be impetuous, and it may even be guarded; on the third or fourth occasion, however, one begins to make progress. As a method of social investigation the free interview in these conditions has something to commend it.

4

This report is mainly about student nurses, although it makes reference also to patients. It has little to say about the methods and technicalities of nursing education, which is a vast subject and no member of the team was qualified to contribute much to its literature. We have, however, reached this conclusion: whereas it may be sufficient, in order to teach French to Tommy, to understand Tommy as well as French, it is imperative that, to teach nursing to Shirley, the ward sister must understand not only both nursing and Shirley; she must also understand herself and her relations with others in the hospital, particularly with the medical and senior nursing staff. In our view, the problems of hospital education have little to do with clinical techniques nor with the formalities and etiquettes in which they are enshrouded; they have, on the other hand, everything to do with the personal relations that spring up between the teachers and the taught. And these in turn are strongly influenced, in our view, by the relation of the teacher to her own nursing superiors and to the doctors under whom she works, and above all, by the extent to which she perceives the hospital as a whole attentive to her own needs and to their satisfaction.

These may be old sentiments; they may have been uttered by voices louder and more commanding than ours; they may even have formed the basis of training policy in some hospitals. Every important nursing conference has much to say upon the subject of human relations and upon the need to bring into hospital training a more humane and sympathetic approach to the student nurse; in our view, any lack of sympathy occasionally displayed by those in authority does not so much derive from defects in their personalities, as from anxiety based on lack of understanding, upon imperfect information, or even upon the misconception of their professional roles. These in turn, derive from inadequate communication, which is both cause and product of unfavourable attitudes. Changes in these cannot be secured merely by speeches from platforms nor by the reported conclusions of research workers. Perhaps the development in the long history of nursing most needed during the next decade is the recognition throughout the profession that techniques—even techniques of communication, such as joint consultation, ward conferences or rapid reading—are of little avail when the real obstructions remain deeply in human attitude and human motive. In a setting as emotional as the ward it will perhaps always remain as necessary as it is convenient to rely upon the standard formula, the agreed procedure, the impersonal and established method. But the integration of the student nurse into the ward team is not merely an exhibition of formalized technique, of ready-made method and of teachable fact; it is no less concerned with the alleviation of her fears and other misgivings, however unreasonable these may seem to those who have been taught by experience consciously to disregard their own. Emotional support plays a part no less than clinical instruction, and such support is of use only if it is offered when it is felt by the student to be needed. It is interesting to observe in some hospitals, where relations are free and formal, that the amount of support and consultation may even appear excessive; a nurse thoroughly at home in her work will nevertheless eagerly discuss her patients with other nurses, and invite their comments upon the way in which she is treating them. Given an atmosphere in which the staff are not discouraged from approaching each other when they feel so inclined, they will go to great lengths to make sure that they are getting the best advice, or, alternatively, most widely distributing the burden of decision, should there be uncertainty about the best course of action to pursue. In a climate of complete relaxation, one may even observe the senior voluntarily consulting the junior about actions that are unequivocally the province of the senior to decide upon; such is the deep need for those who carry the responsibility for human life to feel that they are supported by those around them. It is no wonder that the novices find their lives intolerable when in less permissive conditions, they are denied these fortifying contacts. To those who dismiss the hesitations of the beginner as congenital inadequacies of character that must disqualify her from ever becoming a satisfactory nurse, we may encourage self-examination by quoting the medical authority of St Luke: 'And when He was demanded of the Pharisees, when the Kingdom of God should come, He answered them and said "The Kingdom of God cometh not with observation; neither shall they say, Lo here! or, lo there! for behold, the Kingdom of God is within you"' (Luke, xvii., 20, 21).

In the incident-ridden life of the ward, the most obvious truths may be the most readily forgotten. A professional ethic assuming that neither doctor nor nurse shall become emotionally involved in the patients invariably makes it difficult, and not seldom impossible, for those in authority in the hospital to sense the impression that they make upon those beginners not yet cauterized in the flames of clinical experience. In a profession where 40 per cent of ward sisters (see chapter 7) feel that their own doctors, by rejecting the sisters' suggestions, also depreciate their hard-earned professional experience, what chance have the first-year nurses of catching the sympathetic attention of their ward superiors? Or, by the same token, what can be the expectations of the patient? If the attitude of the doctor is such as to undervalue the experience of the ward-sister and thereby to discourage the interest of the student nurse, what vital information about the patient may the doctor prevent himself from gaining? Might not this discouragement gratuitously add to the uncertainties of the bedside situation, and so both magnify the anxieties of the student and retard the recovery of the patient? Might it not be that the first need is to remove the obstructions unknowingly introduced by the attitude of the doctor? If we may quote again from St Luke: 'And He said unto them, "Ye will surely say unto me this proverb, Physician, heal thyself; whatsoever we have done in Capernaum, do also here in thy country"' (Luke, iv, 23). For this reason, only those who serve in senior situations at the hospital can help it to change, to adapt and to cooperate; if we have learned one thing, it is to seek at least one source of friction in those, whether consultant, matron or administrator, who too readily blame others for the difficulties with which the hospital seems encumbered. The administration is, or should be, that organ of the hospital enabling it to adjust to its environment and this adjustment must embrace the continual solving of the hospital's internal problems; before any person sets out to list the shortcomings of another, he will do well to ask to what extent these are the fruits of a frustration engendered by the critic's own failure to help the person he condemns. Above all, the troubles that accumulate at the lower levels of the hospital and that torment the young nurse during her adjustment to life upon the ward can never be removed by externally imposed changes in syllabus, nor by the temptations of generous pay, nor by other administrative action. Cultural patterns, traditional beliefs, and even personal canons of conduct: all are involved, and all may need amendment. The need for such changes seems, in some hospitals, no less imperative among the committee members than it is among some of the professional staffs themselves; a matron unsupported by her own committee cannot support her sisters. But whether or not it is possible by taking thought and action to change the outlook of so complex a social organism as a hospital is not yet established. The evidence in this study suggests that each hospital has a personality, a character of its own, and that this is largely the expression of its internal stresses and anxieties; not seldom this character forbids the easy assimilation of the new member of the staff, whether student nurse or senior sister. Our thesis is that such a community may be made whole only by itself, by those who work in it. There is no Ministry of Health prototype, no external example, no textbook model, no Platonic ideal, on which it can be fashioned; there is no perfection to be brought about by administrative decree or departmental order alone; those who serve the hospital must perceive their own problems by their own lights and work out their own solutions in their own ways. Whether or not we can suggest any action by which any particular social organism may become more self-aware, and whether, having made these suggestions, we can engineer improvements, remains to be seen. Perhaps it is sufficient to say this: the progress of medical technology over the past century has been such that the internal problems of decision-taking and information-handling in general hospitals are doubling every decade. Moreover, the demand that the patient's treatment shall succeed has also become more imperative. We are required to think of ward situations a hundred times as complicated and exacting as those faced in the reign of Victoria. The student nurse today must be helped to solve problems of learning and adjustment a hundred times as difficult and insistent as those confronting Mrs Wardroper's long-forgotten pioneers; the need for sympathetic consultation between those who console and care for the patient, on the one hand, and those who diagnose and prescribe for him, on the other, is of an order unimaginable to the silk-hatted authoritarians who, from the walls of so many hospital board rooms, look down with haughty disapproval upon a generation that, if less self-satisfied, is also less self-assured. At today's intensity of clinical treatment the problems of hospital administration, in the widest sense of that expression, can no longer be left, as it were, to a small bureaucracy, in the manner that problems of, say, hospital purchasing may still safely be left to one or two professionals. All who work on the ward are caught up in its information and diagnostic network, even if merely to answer a telephone or to indent for a pair of cot sides, and in both of these an untutored girl can make and suffer for her mistakes. If we are to provide the security of understanding essential to those who carry the responsibility in our hospitals, or indeed in any of our social institutions, while the pace of technology is mounting as it is and as it increasingly will, we must understand how people in different stations perceive each other's objectives and each other's problems as readily as we rely upon the help that we expect them to offer, for it is the divergence between these perceptions that endows each hospital with its own peculiar social climate. Indeed, the condition of conflict and confusion arising from the misconception of what others are supposed to know and to do has now been given a name by the anthropologists: parataxis. In our experience the cure for this distressing social malady is the cooperation of those who suffer from it, in solving or in trying to solve some problem in which they are commonly involved; those who successfully tackle one problem together also learn how to deal more readily with the second, and, perhaps, how to prevent a third from ever arising. To learn how common problems may be identified and solved may demand new methods of social investigation, and our report suggests what some of these might be.

1. A comparative study of student nurse wastage

The failure to complete their three years of training and to gain their certificate of State Registration of about half the girls in Britain who become student nurses is a considerable social problem. Many enquiries into this have been reported, but none seems to have asked whether or not the failure rate is significantly greater in some hospitals than in others, and if so, whether it may be influenced by forces under the control of those in charge of the individual hospitals. Comparisons of one hospital with another are, of course, notoriously difficult, for although hospitals are about the most universal of all social institutions they differ as much among themselves as do human individuals, and at first sight comparison of one hospital with another may seem unpromising. Yet differences between human faces, while of importance, say, to those about to get married or to judges of beauty competitions, do not deter students of surface anatomy; although the expressions on the face of any one person may vary from minute to minute, and although the features of one person differ markedly from those of another, there is an underlying uniformity in their anatomical structure upon which the neuro-surgeon can confidently rely.

It is, therefore, of interest to select some hospitals which are reasonably comparable in size, type and social setting, and to examine their statistics of student nurse wastage and of other signs of adjustment to their work. We have chosen five comparable hospitals of industrial Lancashire, and over a period of five years studied how they have managed to deal with their potential nurses. The five hospitals are all designated Class A (acute or mainly acute); all are in towns strictly comparable in the light of such indices as the distribution of population by social class according to the Registrar General; all the towns are, within a few pence, comparable by rateable value per head of population and also by size; all the hospitals are managed by the same Regional Board and, as far as like can be compared with like, we are entitled to compare these hospitals with each other.

We are interested mainly in the reasons why girls abandon their training of their own free will, or of what would be described as their own free will. We therefore divide the total entrants into three classes:

(a) those who successfully complete their training and secure their Certificate of State Registration;
(b) those who withdraw from their training upon their own initiative except to get married; and

9

(c) those who leave the training course for any other reason whatever.

Class (a) above needs no further description. Class (b), although it excepts girls who leave to be married, includes all who otherwise withdraw of their own free will, such as those who say they do not like nursing, who feel that the work is too hard, who are emigrating with their families, and so forth; so long as the motivation comes from the girl, her leaving is recorded in class (b). Class (c) includes all those who are rejected by the hospital either because they fail examinations, or are regarded as unsuitable on grounds of temperament or discipline; it includes all girls who must give up nursing because they are ill; it includes all girls who leave to get married. Using this classification we may set out the statistics for the five hospitals in Table 1.1.

Table 1.1
Total number of student nurses who entered, who completed training—class (a); who withdrew on their own account—class (b); and who left for all other reasons, including marriage—class (c); for five comparable hospitals over five years, 1950–55*

Student nurse	Hospital				
	A	B	C	D	E
Class (a)	197	65	140	103	110
Class (b)	44	21	80	79	146
Class (c)	78	25	38	57	50
Total entries	319	111	258	239	306

* Since the course lasts three years the epoch stretches from 1 January 1950–31 December 1958.

Table 1.1 shows clearly that the incidence of class (b) varies very significantly between hospitals. It is as low as 14 per cent in hospital A, and as high as 48 per cent in hospital E, where we were told it was not unknown for every single girl who entered a particular set (or quarterly entry into the Preliminary Training School) to have given up nursing within a year. The range, in other words, is about 34 per cent, the difference between the highest and the lowest rates. On the other hand, class (c) is much more consistent between these five hospitals and varies only between 15 per cent and 25 per cent, a range of 10 per cent. It is possible to show that this variation is barely significant. Hence we might conclude from this sample that in trying to understand the wide variations between hospitals in their ability to keep their student nurses, it would be our first duty to examine with particular care the reasons given for voluntary withdrawal.

If, indeed, the girls who leave the hospital of their own free will, whatever the ostensible reason they give, do so because they are in fact ill-adjusted to hospital life, we might expect this to show in their sickness-absence records. These are set out in Table 1.2, giving the percentage absence in the five hospitals and for each of the three classes. We see that in each hospital the highest rate of sickness-absence appears among those who have later given up nursing of their own free will. In making these comparisons we have excluded from class (c) the few girls who were obliged to give up nursing because of ill-health. We are here comparing the sickness records of the girls who withdrew voluntarily with those of the girls who either completed their training or who left for all reasons other than ill-health. The chance of the class (b) girls having the worst record in five hospitals without there being an association of sickness with voluntary withdrawal is less than 1 per cent. This result suggests what might be expected, namely, that coming events cast their shadows before them, and that the girls who are eventually to fail in adjusting themselves to life in the hospital show evidence of stress in their sickness patterns before they finally rationalize their withdrawal from training. If this is so and it is claimed that the five hospitals and the girls who enter them are otherwise comparable, it might be argued that

Table 1.2

Percentage sickness-absence rates for three classes of student nurses referred to in Table 1.1.

Student nurse	Hospital				
	A	B	C	D	E
Class (a)	2·51	2·82	3·72	3·78	2·66
Class (b)	4·38	3·75	6·68	6·44	5·47
Class (c)*	2·45	2·47	5·63	4·15	2·96

* Class (c) now excludes all girls who left because of ill-health.

hospitals D and E ought to show worse sickness records than hospital C; in fact they appear to be better. The evidence is that girls are actively discouraged from *reporting sick* at hospitals D and E; this may do something to explain their high wastage rates. A note upon this appears as Appendix 1 (page 81).

It may be said that the differences between sickness rates of different hospitals and of different classes of student nurses within these hospitals depend upon factors that have nothing to do with the adjustment of the girls to their work and training on the wards. It may be objected that we are, after all, comparing the wastage and the sickness-absence of girls in different towns and different hospitals, and thereby ignoring, for example, important local factors, such as climate. We therefore examined the sickness patterns of 600 other girls when serving in another set of hospitals. We could do this because a group of hospitals with a common training scheme arrange that their student nurses serve alternately in different hospitals within the same training group. Its preliminary training school (PTS) is in the main hospital and the student nurses, after spending three months in the school, and three months in the main hospital, then alternate between the other hospitals of the group and the main hospital. Not all girls follow exactly the same series of alternations; some will spend six months or even longer in a single spell at either the main or one of the ancillary hospitals. Nevertheless we may estimate, for all the students who enter this scheme at regular intervals throughout a given period (here two years) and pass completely through it, the average sickness during any particular stage of their training period. Some students will make as many as ten changes during their three years, that is, they will serve, in addition to their three months in the preliminary training school, five times in the main hospital and five times at one or more of the ancillary hospitals. The majority, however, will make no more than seven changes, that is, after their three months in the preliminary training school they will serve for four spells in the main hospital and three in one or more of the ancillaries. Table 1.3 gives the figures for the complete entry of about 600 girls over two years.

Table 1.3 shows that, in the preliminary training school or any of the ancillary hospitals, the sickness-absence rate of the girls is significantly lower than during their service in the main hospital. Sickness-absence has two dimensions: the number of absences per 1000 days at risk and the mean length of the spell once absent. In each case the main hospital is always worse than the ancillary hospitals. There is something about the main hospital which causes the student nurses to be more frequently sick when they serve in it, and which delays their return to work once they have fallen sick. These results are shown graphically in Fig. 1.1 and the differences are very highly significant.

Table 1.3

Sickness-absence statistics for approximately 600 student nurse entrants passing between one main and three ancillary hospitals linked in a common training scheme over two calendar years.

Stage	Where served	No. of days served	No. of days sick	No. of sickness spells	Spells per 1000 days		Mean length of spell (days)	
1	PTS	43 371	310	61	1·41		5·1	
2	Main	53 787	1 141	113		2·11		10·1
3	Anc.	24 723	275	43	1·74		6·4	
4	Main	32 401	943	78		2·41		12·1
5	Anc.	21 799	343	36	1·65		9·5	
6	Main	26 933	1 280	73		2·72		17·5
7	Anc.	14 933	178	26	1·75		6·8	
8	Main	25 362	972	65		2·56		15·0
9	Anc.	6 577	64	10	1·52		6·4	
10	Main	13 342	541	36		2·70		15·0
11	Anc.	1 782	15	3	1·69		5·0	

In preparing this table any sickness-absence that began while the student was on leave in an interval between changing hospitals has been omitted. If a student nurse went directly from one ancillary hospital to another, her days served and sickness-absence are attributed to the same joint ancillary stage.

Figure 1.1 Nurses in training at hospital, M, and associated institutions, A.

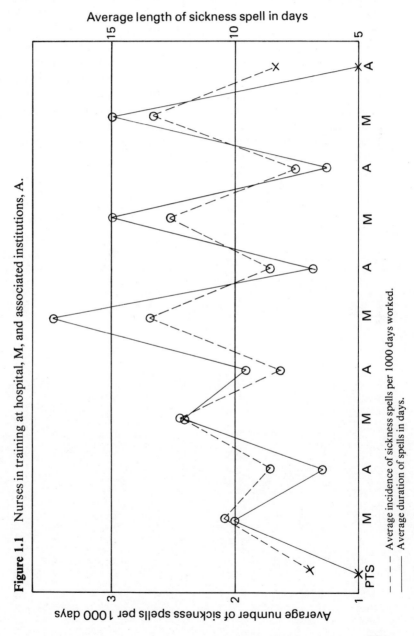

Average length of sickness spell in days

Average number of sickness spells per 1000 days

--- Average incidence of sickness spells per 1000 days worked.
— Average duration of spells in days.

13

Table 1.3 and Fig. 1.1 not only put beyond all doubt the suggestion that the differences between the sickness rates of student nurses are significant, but a comparison of the main hospital with the ancillaries suggests at least one precipitating cause. The main hospital is much larger than the ancillary hospitals; in interview the student nurses who passed through the scheme observed that the size of the main hospital and its pace of work made it comparatively difficult for them to understand what was going on. We may suggest from this that the extent to which the student nurse finds her work to be intelligible is at least an indication of her security; where she feels that she may, beyond a reasonable limit, be expected to take responsibility for matters that she cannot understand, there is a significant likelihood that she will first fall ill, and later even abandon her training. The extent to which the hospital can bring this intelligibility to the nurses who serve on its wards must, other things being equal, depend upon its size and there is evidence, apart from that above, to suggest that large hospitals have peculiar problems of their own. Two unusual examples of the stresses of large hospitals are given in Appendix 2 (page 82).

2. The adjustment of other hospital staff

If the responses of the student nurses to their experiences in the several Lancashire hospitals are so different, it is reasonable to ask whether other classes of nurse also display responses that differ significantly from one hospital to another. It is more difficult to answer this simple question than might at first be imagined, since hospitals in general have no tradition of personnel management, and their records are not usually in a form that makes comparison of one hospital with another a simple affair. Nevertheless, in the five hospitals at which the student nurse wastage was examined, it was possible, after the expenditure of nearly one whole year of effort on the part of a research student, to tabulate the periods of service of nearly 6000 women who, to some extent, shared the experiences of the student nurses.

These women were of several different classes; matrons and their deputies, ward sisters, staff nurses, assistant nurses and domestics. Matrons and their deputies do not, of course, join in the tasks of the ward with the student nurses; many of the domestics never go on the wards. There are, however, four classes of nurse—ward sister, staff nurse, assistant nurse and student—who work, or should work, closely as a team; it might be expected that, in any one hospital, the wastage or retention patterns of the four classes were significantly concordant.

Table 2.1 gives the distribution, by hospital and by category, of the mean period of stay in months, of 5828 women at the five hospitals and in the six employment categories. One category totals only 35 members, the matrons and deputy matrons at the five hospitals, over the years 1938–56 inclusive; the other categories give the figures for 1949–56 inclusive.

It can be shown that the array of Table 2.1 has a highly significant concordance. We may, for example, write the average periods of stay of the four ward categories of nurse in rank order and obtain Table 2.2.

This table suggests that hospitals A and B are consistently better than any others and that D and E are generally bad. The probability that this could occur at random is about once in a thousand times; we must thus conclude that the tendencies of hospitals A and B to keep their ward staff and of hospitals D and E not to do so are organic. If, in addition to the four classes of women who work together on the wards, we consider the two further classes, of matrons and domestics, the concordance is repeated, so that we are able to assert with confidence that, in any one hospital, there is throughout some factor with which the wastage of all staff is, in some significant degree, associated. If we, for example,

Table 2.1

Average period of stay in months for the five hospitals and six categories of women staff (periods below three days given to nearest tenth part of one month).

		Mean period of stay (months) for given hospital and category					
Hosp.	Turnover of staff at hosp.	Matrons and dp. mt.	Ward sisters	Staff nurses	Asst nurses	Student nurses	Domestic workers
A	979	188	59	12·5	28·3	33·5	30·7
B	792	74	87	14·3	26·0	32·6	16·9
C	1354	150	44	11·8	16·8	30·4	28·6
D	889	44	29·5	9·2	7·1	30·1	21·4
E	1814	101	57	8·5	18·3	27·4	17·4
No. of staff all	5828	35	444	992	575	1233	2549

Table 2.2

Rank order of average length of stay by five hospitals and four categories of ward staff.

Hospitals	Ward sisters	Staff nurses	Assistant nurses	Student nurses
A	2	2	1	1
B	1	1	2	2
C	4	3	4	3
D	5	4	5	4
E	3	5	3	5

contrast the averages of hospitals A and D in Table 2.1, we obtain the two series of ranks:

Hospital A: first, second, second, first, first, first
Hospital D: fifth, fifth, fourth, fifth, fourth, third.

A man who, after reading the results of six successive appearances of two racehorses or of two beauty queens, discovered that they had been ranked in these orders, would have no doubt whatever that there was a reason for the consistent ascendancy of A over D. He would refuse to admit (unless he was grossly biased by, say, owning the losing racehorse or being married to the rejected beauty queen) that the results were purely random; he would, on the contrary, say they were *caused*, either, in the one event, by A being a faster racehorse or, in the other, by A's more evident, if superficial, attractions for the kind of men who judge women by their appearance.

The importance of this result is to remove any suggestion that the wastage of student nurses at any particular hospital is, as it were, something on its own, a localized or specific symptom to be treated independently of the general state of staff wastage throughout the hospital as a whole. It may, of course, very well be that one can profitably prescribe treatment specific to student nurse wastage, such as to change the conditions under which they are taught in the training school; such therapy might not react much upon the rest of the hospital staff. But if one attempted to improve the conditions under which they were, say, taught on the wards, one might begin to put right matters of importance to other grades of staff as well. It is, on the other hand, conceivable that, in trying to improve certain limited conditions for one class of nurse, conditions may be made worse for another, though in practice this is unlikely. If, for example, ward sisters protested loudly enough, for long enough, that they had no privileges in securing time off on desirable occasions (such as Saturday afternoons) but were obliged to await their turn with their juniors, it might eventually be conceded that they were given priority for off-duty hours. This would, however, suggest favouritism to others on the ward and might have an unhappy effect upon their loyalty to the hospital. But such inverse interactions would be rare; in general, as Table 2.2 suggests, whatever strengthens the attachment of one group to the hospital undoubtedly strengthens the attachment of others.

The relevance of this result should be apparent. For when it is pointed out to the administrators of some hospitals that the wastage rate among their student nurses is higher than the regional average, their first reaction is to attribute this to the ease with which the fugitives are able to secure interesting or lucrative employment in the locality. Since the girls who leave can be observed to have taken work somewhere in local offices, mills or retail stores, and since it is improbable that they would be paid less than as nurses, it is often asserted that high wages or short hours have seduced them from the arduous toil of the wards; their romantic yearnings are now satisfied, it is explained, and they are awakened to reality. But ward sisters, much less matrons, do not leave hospitals in order to earn high wages in easy jobs at local shops or factories; they give up their posts at particular hospitals in order to seek conditions more agreeable to them in other hospitals. Many student nurses would wish to follow their example, but are at times unable to do so—or believe themselves unable to do so—because, it is said, matrons in charge of training schools are reluctant to take on student nurses who fail, for whatever reason, to complete their training at other hospitals. We have no evidence other than the statements of the student nurses for this. However this may be, the simple demonstration that the wastage patterns of all grades of nursing staff in the same hospital show this concordance should be enough to discredit any explanation of wastage that assumes the student nurses to be, as a singular class, dragged from the hospital by outside attractions rather than motivated to leave it by internal pressures felt also by their more senior colleagues on the same wards.

A further argument against the young girls in certain towns being positively attracted by other work may be built upon the employment statistics. For example, we can ask how long girls of the same age as student nurses stay in other jobs in the three towns of hospitals A, C and E; if the high wastage at hospital E is encouraged by a high local availability of easy and well-paid jobs and the retentivity of hospital A by the comparative absence of such opportunities, with hospital C in between, we might anticipate some reflection on this in the local employment statistics. We were fortunate, in trying to answer this question, to get the help of a nationally known chain store that takes a great deal of trouble to select and train its staff, most of whom begin as girls of the same age as nurses. Over the same five-year period as that chosen in chapter 1 to examine the wastage of the student nurses, the figures for recruitment and wastage in the chain stores of the three towns are as given in Table 2.3 together with the percentage of voluntary wastage among the student nurses.

Table 2.3

Number of employees on books over a period of five years and mean length of stay in employment for three stores belonging to the same organization; and, for comparison, percentage voluntary wastage of student nurses from hospitals in the same town over the same period.

Town of hospital	Number of employees	Av. period of employment	Av. voluntary nurse wastage
A	174	5y 2m	14%
C	232	2y 2m	31%
E	154	5y 0m	48%

It can be seen that there is no significant difference in the responses of the store girls in the towns of hospitals A and E; these two hospitals, on the contrary, display marked differences in their abilities to retain the student nurses they recruit. Moreover, whereas the mean wastage of student nurses in hospital C is exactly the average of hospitals A and E together, the turnover of staff in the local store is more than double that of the stores in the towns of hospitals A and E. We have, on examining other aspects of employment in these towns, been able to find no evidence that it is easier to change jobs in the town of hospital E than in the others, and must therefore conclude once more that external conditions cannot be invoked to explain the significant differences between the attachments of student nurses to their respective hospitals.

3. The length of patient stay

These studies of student nurse wastage and sickness and of the loss of other nursing and domestic staff in a number of hospitals suggest that there is, of any given hospital, some characteristic helping significantly to determine the willingness of the staff to stay in its service. Hospitals that cannot keep junior nurses tend not to keep ward sisters; they do not readily keep domestics, and they seem unable to keep even their matrons. We must ask whether these same hospital qualities are likely to influence the observable experiences of the patients. In the present state of our knowledge the simplest way of approaching this question is to ask if the average length of patient stay differs significantly from one hospital to another, and, if so, whether it is likely to do so for reasons internal to the hospital and so, perhaps, under the control of those who serve there. Insofar as we have been able to make use of the statistical evidence available to us, the answers to this question are, first, that hospitals differ significantly in their average lengths of patient stay, that hospitals keeping one diagnostic group of patient longer than average tend to keep other groups longer, and that hospitals with unstable nursing staffs tend to return long periods of patient stay in all specialties.

The first survey, involving the examination of some 3000 case notes, was undertaken in seven acute general hospitals, all situated in large towns in the North of England. The patient specialties studied were all surgical: appendicectomy, hernia repair, cholecystectomy and partial gastrectomy.

These four diagnoses were chosen, in the first instance, as offering reasonably large numbers of cases with a consistent average length of stay; they were each studied in all seven hospitals over a period of one year, namely, 1959. Care has thus been taken to ensure that the inter-hospital comparisons are meaningful and that the results are significant, even although sampling has taken place.

The use of convalescent homes attracted attention early in the survey. At one extreme was the hospital which does not use convalescent homes at all, mainly due to their remoteness or restricted availability; at the other extreme was the hospital which sends 70 per cent of its general surgery patients to convalescent homes before discharge. We found, as one would expect, that patients who also go to a convalescent home spend a shorter time in the hospital itself, but a total time away from home longer than of those who are treated wholly in the hospital. For strict comparisons between hospitals, only those patients wholly treated in the hospital itself have been considered here. It is assumed that the availability or otherwise of a convalescent home does not alter the treatment accorded to 'hospital-only' patients.

We studied the records of 654 appendicectomies, with a mean stay of approximately 10 days; about half of the cases (331) have lengths of stay of 7, 8 or 9 days, with an extreme range from 2 to 56 days. The layman and, not seldom, the doctor may feel that, because the data are so variable, that is, because there is this great spread, no useful conclusions may be drawn. On the contrary, when presented with a mass of variable data which can be classified, the statistician may be able to say that a measurable amount of the variation is due to differences between the classes, and the remaining variation is due to differences within them. Here we can say that the variation of the 654 lengths of stay is due to both real differences in average length of stay between hospitals and also the variation in lengths of stay of individual patients in each hospital about that hospital average.

The results of the inter-hospital comparisons for the appendicectomies are given in Table 3.1. The differences in numbers of cases are due not only to the varying sizes of hospital but also to the extent to which each hospital uses its convalescent home, since patients sent to convalescent homes do not contribute to our analysis.

Table 3.1

Average length of stay of appendicectomy cases not using convalescent homes in the seven hospitals.

Hospital	Number of cases under consideration	Mean length of stay in days
I	153	8·3
II	45	8·8
III	66	10·8
IV	93	11·6
V	150	11·1
VI	74	10·7
VII	73	9·6
Total	654	10·11

It can be shown (see Appendix 3, page 85) that these averages differ significantly between themselves, that is, the differences between them cannot be accounted for by the variations in length of stay of individual patients. The mean of hospital IV is 40 per cent more than the mean of hospital I; the chance of this being due to sampling is much less than one in a million. Nor can we invoke differences between the pressures on the hospitals from the waiting lists; indeed, hospitals with long waiting lists often had the longest periods of patient stay and vice versa. This situation would be perfectly intelligible to a student of queueing theory, which demonstrates that given equal demand, the mean length of queue depends upon the service time. Hospitals, of course, do not entirely present random queueing situations, since many patients are advised when to come for admission; the analogy, however, is not misleading.

This analysis can be carried one stage further. Any patient is treated under one and only one of a group of consultants, each of whom normally uses a specific ward or wards. Thus it could be argued that variation in individual lengths of stay is partly due to significant differences between the practices or policies of the consultants. We can test this by classifying patients in any hospital by the consultant responsible, and once more examining the interclass variations. There were, for example, four general surgical consultants in hospital I, and the results of these inter-consultant comparisons are shown in Table 3.2.

Table 3.2

Average length of stay of appendicectomies treated by four different consultants in hospital I.

Consultant	No. of cases treated	Av. length of stay in days
(a)	28	8·8
(b)	47	8·1
(c)	23	8·5
(d)	55	8·1

These differences are not significant, that is to say, variations in individual lengths of stay cannot be assigned to differences between consultants. These conclusions for appendicectomy cases hold for each of the three other diagnostic groups at hospital I. When the appendicectomies in the other six hospitals are examined for possible consultant differences, the same conclusion is found. The data have also been analysed for possible differences due to the ward used and any differences so reflected could be attributed to differences between sexes, women tending to remain significantly longer than men. Similar results also apply in each of the three other groups of cases; that is, consultants and wards in any one hospital show no differences among themselves. We may therefore conclude that some factor characteristic of a given hospital seems to influence the time which any individual patient stays in it, whatever his diagnostic group, whoever his consultant and whatever his ward.

This examination of the case notes leads us to search for the characteristics of particular hospitals. We may ask a further question: if one hospital takes longer to discharge comparable surgical patients, does it also take longer to prepare them for their operations? The evidence is set out in Table 3.3, which shows in its left-hand array the rank order, for the seven hospitals and the four conditions, of the average length of pre-operation period.

Table 3.3

Rank orders of average pre-operation and post-operation periods for seven general hospitals and four common surgical diagnoses.

Hospital	Rank order of average length of period							
	pre-operation				post-operation			
	A	*H*	*C*	*G*	*A*	*H*	*C*	*G*
I	6	4	4	2	3	1	1	5
II	5	5	6	3	7	6	5	6
III	7	7	7	7	6	7	6	7
IV	3	3	3	4	5	4	3	2
V	1	6	5	6	2	2	7	3
VI	2	2	2	5	1	3	2	1
VII	4	1	1	1	4	5	4	4

A. appendicectomy   H. hernia repair
C. cholecystectomy   G. partial gastrectomy

The coefficient of concordance of this left-hand array is 0·60, significant at one part in a hundred. In other words, on the evidence of 3000 surgical cases in seven general hospitals, drawn from four common operation classes, we may assert with confidence that hospitals that are slow to prepare one class of patient are slow to prepare another. Since, in any one hospital, there seems to be no difference between the patterns of the individual surgeons in that hospital, we may conclude that the validity of our hypothesis about hospital characteristics has been further demonstrated. We may draw the same conclusion from the right-hand array of Table 3.3, which ranks the average periods between operation and discharge. This array demonstrates, again at a significance level of one in a hundred, that the hospital at which one patient is rapidly discharged after operation for appendicectomy tends rapidly to discharge after operation another patient for hernia repair, and so forth. Finally, if the two arrays are considered together, they show greater concordance still; the random chance, for example, of the total rank-score of hospital III amounting to as much as 54 (suggesting slowness throughout) while that of hospital VI is as little as 18 (suggesting swiftness throughout) is less than 1 in 1000. Despite the apparent scatter in this table (hospital V, for example, being top of the list on one score and bottom on another) it suggests a consistency about the velocity of patient treatment in individual hospitals such as should merit the attention of students of their administration.

While this essay was being written, a set of statistics from a report prepared by the statistician to a Regional Hospital Board came into our hands. They included figures, for average length of patient stay, prepared by hospital staffs to whom the arguments of this chapter must be unknown; they may thus be used for an independent test of this hypothesis. The set of figures was for 34 hospitals and for nine diagnostic groups; some hospitals did not admit patients in certain groups, others used the services of convalescent units. An array of average lengths of stay by hospitals and by all diagnostic groups is prepared to satisfy the following conditions:

(a) no hospital selected shall use a convalescent unit, so that all patients are discharged home and thus, in comparing average stays, like is being compared with like;

(b) the number of patients in any diagnostic group in any hospital in the period (1961) shall be at least 12;

and this is shown at Table 3.4; it is drawn for 14 hospitals and for nine diagnostic groups. The other 20 hospitals either discharged to convalescent units or did not admit enough patients in any diagnostic group. The coefficient of concordance of this array is 0.37 and is very highly significant; the tendency for the shorter stays to appear in particular hospitals and the longer stays in other hospitals could not possibly have occurred by chance (see Appendix 4, page 86). We may thus assert with confidence that there is some hospital factor associated with shortness or length of stay. This is not likely to be pressure upon beds, since there was no correlation whatever by hospitals between mean bed occupancy and mean length of stay. Nor is it helpful to suggest that some administrative artefact such as a systematic difference between admission and operation days could explain this concordance. If one hospital, to take an extreme case, admitted patients only on Mondays and discharged only on Fridays (always, moreover, keeping the patients longer rather than discharging sooner) the mean length of stay would be about three days greater than in the hospital giving identical treatment but discharging at any time during the week. Six of the nine ranges in Table 3.4 exceed a week.

We know very little about the final decision to discharge a patient from hospital, and until all the events that lead up to it have been examined in a wide sample, drawn from different hospitals, different consultants, different wards and different patients, we shall continue to know very little. What these hospital factors contribute we do not know, although we may make interesting guesses. Perhaps in an age of advancing medical and surgical technology, some hospitals are slow, not so much to use current methods, as to show confidence in their results; for this reason patients, although getting the same benefits as those in other hospitals, are retained as long as formerly, 'just in case'. Perhaps the patients in fact recover more slowly; nobody is surprised when two 'identical' patients in adjacent beds improve at significantly different rates, because one liked his nurses and the doctors, while the other found them short-tempered, or too busy to pay much attention to him. Is it not possible that such differences could be detected, not only between individual patients, paired in adjacent beds, but also between large aggregations of patients, paired in adjacent hospitals?

Patient stay and staff wastage

We must now ask whether these hospital characteristics are likely to be associated with the stability of the staff. We set out in Table 3.5 the average

Table 3.4

Mean length of patient stay (in days) in nine diagnostic groups for 14 hospitals in the same region.

Hospital	(a)	(b)	(c)	(d)	(e)	(f)	(g)	(h)	(i)
I	25·0	10·3	11·4	17·6	16·7	15·4	9·1	10·0	13·9
II	27·4	16·5	11·9	12·8	10·8	9·7	9·3	13·3	20·4
III	27·4	15·7	12·6	22·0	17·2	20·3	9·6	11·9	18·2
IV	23·2	14·1	11·7	19·8	23·6	18·8	9·7	10·4	14·8
V	21·6	12·0	12·1	16·6	12·9	16·7	12·2	11·1	17·7
VI	23·9	9·4	9·6	15·6	14·9	13·5	10·6	10·1	11·7
VII	20·4	10·6	10·6	12·6	11·9	15·6	10·7	11·2	16·7
VIII	21·5	11·9	11·8	11·6	12·5	17·0	10·3	12·7	16·8
IX	19·8	8·9	12·6	13·0	14·9	18·8	10·0	11·7	14·7
X	19·2	12·9	10·2	14·6	11·9	16·7	11·6	11·0	18·4
XI	23·9	13·5	11·2	16·9	19·6	17·2	11·4	13·5	19·0
XII	25·8	13·6	12·1	18·5	16·5	20·4	10·5	13·4	19·3
XIII	19·3	21·3	12·9	16·8	12·3	19·4	14·6	10·9	18·6
XIV	16·6	11·1	10·6	13·3	13·6	12·5	10·6	10·6	14·3

(a) arteriosclerotic heart disease
(b) varicose veins
(c) haemorrhoids
(d) pneumonia
(e) bronchitis

(f) peptic ulcer
(g) appendicitis
(h) hernia repair
(i) diseases of gall bladder

lengths of stay for 1958 of five sets of patients at the five hospitals whose staff wastage is discussed in chapter 2; in addition to the four surgical operations of appendicectomy, hernia repair, cholecystectomy and partial gastrectomy, we have included the diagnostic group of respiratory complaints, asthma, bronchitis and pneumonia.

This shows that, in four out of five classes, hospital A has the shortest mean stay, while hospitals D or E have the longest. The concordance, or tendency of

Table 3.5

Average length of stay in days according to diagnostic group for 4752 patients discharged from five comparable Lancashire hospitals.

Hosp.	No. of patients	App.	H.R.	Chol.	P.G.	Resp.
A	1362	7·5	7·9	12·2	15·5	15·7
B	669	9·5	10·9	18·1	17·3	20·0
C	766	10·9	13·1	17·7	15·0	20·1
D	496	11·6	14·0	23·9	27·6	24·0
E	1459	12·1	13·6	26·7	26·1	20·6
Total no. of cases	4752	2059	894	493	290	1016

the five hospitals to display a uniformity of response independent of the specialty or diagnostic group is so great that it could not occur by chance once in a thousand times. It must therefore, as we argue from Table 3.4, be caused; it is the manifestation of a set of characteristics proper to the five hospitals. Moreover, we can see from Table 3.6, obtained by placing Table 2.2 of chapter 2 side by side with Table 3.5 (converted to rankings rather than averages expressed in days), that the concordance of patient stay is probably that of staff stability as well.

Table 3.6
Rank orders of staff and patient stay for five comparable hospitals.

Hosp.	Rank orders of staff stay				Rank orders of patient stay				
	ward sister	staff nurse	asst nurse	student nurse	App.	H.R.	Chol.	P.G.	Resp.
A	2	2	1	1	1	1	1	2	1
B	1	1	2	2	2	2	3	3	2
C	4	3	4	3	3	3	2	1	3
D	5	4	5	4	4	5	4	5	5
E	3	5	3	5	5	4	5	4	4

This table aligns the stability of the ward nursing staff with the average period of patient stay; the concordance throughout the two arrays is overwhelming. If the tendency for hospital A to attract the small numbers and hospital D the large is purely random, we are observing the occurrence of an event that could occur at random (that is, without underlying cause) not once in a million times. It is impossible to overlook the chance that the two sets of figures, of patient stay and of ward staff stay, might be causally related. For if there is some quality about a hospital ward, or about all the wards in a particular hospital, that determines the desire of those who work there to get away (or to stay) it is inconceivable that the patients should be unaffected by this quality, whatever its nature or origins. We obviously cannot identify it by further statistical analysis alone; it is essential to study the situations on the wards, and in this the following quotation, from the writings of a research worker who, independently of this study, interviewed many hundreds of recently discharged patients, may offer a suggestion.

'The importance of the ward sister to the patient cannot be over-emphasized. The junior nurse would be judged perhaps by her friendliness, a staff nurse perhaps by her technical skill, but the ward sister was judged by the atmosphere of the ward. This, if its importance can be judged by the number of times it was mentioned, was of the utmost importance to patients, some of whom claimed a direct correlation between the rate of recovery and the atmosphere of the ward.' (*The Patient's Attitude to Nursing Care*, Anne McGhee, page 41.) The main thesis of this essay could not have been more lucidly stated.

4. The analysis of ward activities

To anticipate the results of our detailed studies on the wards we may say here that the student nurse has two main needs: the first is to acquire adequate technical knowledge of her job and the second is to establish herself as a person. She needs not only clinical instruction but emotional support; she has not only to learn how to carry through such-and-such a procedure and be marked up in the record as having done so, but she has also to gain that confidence in herself to carry out that procedure in the face of the recurrent stresses and anxieties of her ward experience; this means that she will have to gain the confidence to enable her to decide the priorities of urgent tasks, or of the claims of equally ill patients. While confidence in one's own ability lends support in all situations, the young nurse also needs to know that in moments of particular stress she can confidently call upon the support of others. When one hears matrons of fifty admit (in a quite different context) that they still feel uneasily inferior discussing some latest circular with their medical colleagues, or even that to face regular meetings with their ward sisters is still a prospect of dread, it is small wonder that, in the first three months of life on the ward (or, more so, in her first week of night duty) the young nurse needs the friendship of those more experienced than herself. A girl in her first year may, in the sense of being able to answer questions formally put at a lesson in a classroom, know as perfectly as does the President of the Royal College of Physicians what should be done in such-and-such a bedside situation. But in the solitary darkness of her first night duty her approach to what needs to be done, of what she knows about it, and of how she does it may be very different from her confident exhibition under the academic cross examination of her sister-tutor; at her first midnight it may be of major importance that the superintendent on duty promptly answers her call, if only to reassure her that she is doing the right thing. We show, for example, that in free interviews the student nurses volunteer more than twice as many comments on interpersonal relations within the hospital as they do about their experiences of formal training (see chapter 6). It is these interpersonal relations in the work situation that determine how far the student regards her new experiences with interest and gratification, or how far, on the contrary, they are sources of anxiety or even of loss of self-respect.

In order to understand how far the nurse finds support in her new responsibilities we need to know how far the sister in charge of the ward is able to spend time with the new recruit, and how far those formally in charge of nurse training are able to give general supervision to her integration into the hospital. We must answer at least two questions: What are the relations between the ward sisters and the sister-tutor? How does the ward sister spend her time?

We do not propose to say a great deal about the first of these, except that these relations vary greatly between hospitals. We found, for example, that about half the ward sisters interviewed felt that formal training schemes were too theoretical; about a quarter of the sisters thought they actually glamourized the ward task. The strength of these views differed widely between hospitals, but their existence suggests stress between the wards and the training schools. On the other hand, we found the sisters and junior nurses in some hospitals speaking appreciatively of the tutorial staff, although their views of the organization as a whole were extremely unfavourable; in one hospital that could be described only as socially sick (hospital Q of Table 6.1), the nursing staff almost without exception spoke warmly of the training system. Had this been informed by the same unhappy spirit as the rest of the organization the general condition of the hospital would have been sorry indeed; that it was not so may be attributed mainly to the cheerful temperament of one or two of the senior tutorial staff. In other hospitals we found the division between the ward sisters and the tutors such that the sisters were never invited to visit or to lecture in the training school, nor did the sister-tutors ever visit the wards to observe the progress of the students. The study-blocks spent by the student nurses back in the training school, during which they received further instruction from the tutors, were carried on in complete isolation from the ward staff; these, in turn, taught, supervised, and recorded as satisfactorily completed or not, the large number of clinical procedures in which the student must be proficient to gain her registration; and all this was done without the ward sisters being taught how to give a demonstration, how to gauge whether the student nurse is in fact learning, or in any other way how to profit from the professional knowledge at hand in the tutors of the training school. Several hospitals seemed almost determined to preserve this isolation of interest, to keep the ward and the training schools divided, and their plans for new buildings generally assumed that they would remain apart. While it is no doubt possible to attribute some of these antagonisms, along with endless others to be found, alas, in every corner of our institutionalized society, to the infirmities of human nature, it was nonetheless remarkable to discover that the management committees of these hospitals, responsible for their policies, were largely unaware of them. Although they spent a great deal of time discussing the wastage of nurses and its consequences for the staffing of the wards, they were unaware, or appeared to be unaware, of the internecine struggles that went on inside the very training system itself, and that were taken up afresh as one redoubtable generation succeeded another. The current move to appoint clinical tutors to take over the more complex instruction on the wards will, if it is to succeed, often demand all the good will available, and, occasionally, somewhat more. Nor is this all. Some very delicate questions about the responsibility for and supervision of these itinerants will need to be answered; in particular, they cannot pretend to relieve the ward sister of her vital task of lending the student nurse the emotional support that she will so often need.

These examples may be exceptional, but they serve to show some of the effects of the human problems that may arise in the higher levels of the nursing administration itself. If the senior tutor and the ward sisters are not on wholly good terms—and this is primarily a problem for the matron, or in a group scheme for the several matrons—it is the student nurses who suffer. An interesting problem in administration, that will be touched on later, is raised for the hospital management committee: how does it know what in fact goes on, as distinct from what is said to go on, at the point where the student nurses gain experience? The same question may be asked about hospital cadets. The impending concentration of training into the larger general hospitals will make it the more necessary to give attention to these delicate but often opaque affairs. The hospital service has plenty of favourable experience with which to answer these questions; the problem is to bring it to the attention of those who may have such problems without being clearly aware of them. On the other hand, we found one hospital in which there was the greatest good will between the ward staff and the training staff and in which constant experiment was going on to discover what was better taught by the sisters as part of normal ward duty, and what was better done by the clinical tutors drawn into the wards from the training schools. This seems to us the perfect solution to a difficult problem; namely, that the tutors and the ward sisters should not merely agree about how to share out the training task, but that they should from time to time adjust their respective shares. A hospital that constantly reviews its own organization is learning to know itself, and it learns not only about its current problems, but also about its channels of communication, its various informal structures, its status system and, above all, the impact that its staff have upon each other. In our view, one of the greatest needs is that all management committees should encourage amongst their senior professional staffs some such spirit of enquiry and criticism. The good hospitals that we encountered seemed always unafraid, even positively anxious, to discuss their problems; the committees and staffs of the bad ones generally denied that they had any. A concern for what is going on within the hospital, and an awareness of the problems on the wards, are not merely to display some patronizing encouragement calculated to raise the flagging energies of the over-burdened nurses; the problems of many hospitals are both so deeply organic and so ill-perceived by those in positions of power that only by developing internal methods of social learning to make the senior staffs more aware of what is happening under their jurisdiction will there be promise of improvement.

To understand how much attention the ward sister is able to devote to the integration of her student nurses we must know something of the sister's work patterns. It is possible to form an accurate enough estimate of the amount of time that she gives to the four main divisions of her work, namely, administration, basic nursing, technical nursing and domestic and miscellaneous activities. (*The Work of Nurses in Hospital Wards*, London, Nuffield Provincial Hospitals Trust, (1953)). In studying the work of the sisters, the two classes of domestic

28

and miscellaneous separately observed in this earlier Nuffield Report have been amalgamated, since sisters carry out little domestic work as specified by that report.) In this classification, 'administration' includes all those duties of the ward sister that bring her into contact both with other members of her ward team and with other persons in the hospital—doctors, matron, administrative staff, staff of para-medical and ancillary departments, and so forth. Administration, therefore, might be described as 'collecting, processing and transmitting information about the work of the ward'.

A number of observers have developed methods of recording the minute to minute tasks of the sisters and some typical results are given in Table 4.1.

Table 4.1

Percentages of ward time spent on four main classes of activity by seven sisters in one large Manchester hospital.

Sister	Administration	Basic nursing	Technical nursing	Domestic and miscellaneous
A	34	17	41	8
B	36	19	35	10
C	44	18	32	6
D	44	9	29	18
E	26	29	32	13
F	28	21	21	30
G	59	6	20	15

The distribution of how her time is spent varies from one sister to another according, to some extent, to the nature of the work carried out on the ward. Table 4.1, which analyses over 200 hours of activity, is drawn for seven sisters at one particular hospital; judged by the criteria used in this report the hospital was a good one and this particular table is included since sister E was regarded by her matron as a quite exceptional nurse. She had, in fact, some years before sought promotion and become the matron of a small hospital; she had, it was told, been successful at this task; after a short while she had decided that her true calling was with the patients and had returned to her task on the ward at her old hospital. She was respected by all the other nurses to whom we spoke and the students regarded it as a privilege to work for her.

We observe that administration is, averaged over all the sisters, the activity that occupies the greatest share of their time, namely, about 39 per cent; after this comes, as would be expected, technical nursing, averaging 30 per cent, and basic nursing, average 19 per cent. But there is the greatest variety among the individual sisters themselves. Whereas sister E devotes only 26 per cent of her time to administration, sister G devotes 59 per cent; this is a very great difference and there was nothing to suggest that sister G's ward was better organized than sister E's. Indeed, the difference was in favour of sister E. Sister E, we observe,

29

spent significantly more time than her colleagues on basic nursing; she was not surprised when this was pointed out to her and remarked that this probably gave her more opportunity to understand both her patients and her junior nurses, since informal conversation was easier when engaged in simple tasks with her staff than when performing delicate procedures. We notice, however, that she did the average share of technical nursing. Her scores differ markedly in two respects from most of her colleagues, except sister F, in that she spent much less time on administration and considerably more upon basic nursing. Different sisters must, of course, decide for themselves in what ways they will make easy and informal contacts with their juniors, but certainly sharing the tasks of basic nursing with them is as promising an avenue of contact as any other. There is a significant negative correlation between time spent on basic nursing and time spent on administration; sisters who become absorbed in written work spend little time with their students.

Our observations of the ward sister's activities may be sorted in order to exhibit the amount of conversation that she has with her ward team. In general, ward sisters average about ten conversations an hour with all other persons in the hospital, from consultants to porters, from ministers of religion to ward maids; this excludes conversation with patients. Of these ten per hour, about half are with her own subordinates, half with hospital staff elsewhere. For a number of wards that were observed in detail, each for a total period of about 30 hours, a representative distribution of the sister's conversations, by length, with subordinates, by rank, is set out in Table 4.2. These observations were made mostly during the busy morning hours of 8.00 a.m. until 1.00 p.m.

This reveals an average rate of about five conversations per hour. Of these the majority last less than half a minute. It is rare, or it was during these observations in this hospital, for a ward sister to spend more than two minutes in continuous conversation with any of her subordinates; she will, of course, have much longer conversations with her superiors, although they may be less frequent. What is striking is the small amount of time here shown as spent in conversation with the first year nurses. It is clear from this sample of obser-

Table 4.2

Distribution, by length of time and by members of subordinate ward nursing staff, of conversations of ward sisters over approximately 30 hours.

Grade of ward staff	Number and lengths of conversations in minutes					
	0–$\frac{1}{2}$	$\frac{1}{2}$–1	1–2	2–5	5+	all
Junior sister	16	3	2	1	0	22
Staff nurse	31	1	2	3	2	39
3rd year student	40	0	2	2	1	45
2nd year student	37	0	1	0	0	38
1st year student	13	0	0	1	0	14
All	137	4	7	7	3	158

30

vations that, the more senior the nurse (except for the junior sister, who mainly gets on with her tasks without needing to consult her immediate superior), the more time she is able to claim from the sister, and this can be taken to suggest the measure of her usefulness or responsibility in sharing the total task to be done on the ward. Other observations suggest that sisters spend between 5 per cent and 7 per cent of their time in conversation with their subordinate nurses; this is very small compared with the figures suggesting the total amount of their time devoted to administration, namely, from 26 per cent to 59 per cent. The range of this is about six times the average total time devoted to conversation with all her subordinate nurses, and an even greater multiple of the time that she spends in conversation with her first year nurse; in the example given, this is less than 1 per cent of the ward sister's time. Hence the planned or even the adventitious induction of the student nurse must occupy only the most marginal amount of the average ward sister's attention, since over half of the conversations that the sister can be observed to engage in with her are little more than direct instructions and their acknowledgement. They are in no way the exchange of ideas and the sharpening of perception that form the essence of true learning, either by the nurse or by the sister. But when we come to examine the time spent by the ward sisters in other forms of administration we find that some of them spend up to 30 per cent of their time on purely clerical activity. We found, both by these direct observations on the wards, as well as by the commitments to clerical work expressed by the ward sisters, that there were significant differences not only between sisters but also between hospitals. While (as in chapter 7 and Appendix 5) we find no evidence that sisters with deep concern for clerical work actually express attitudes towards junior nurses that are less sympathetic than those who carry this commitment lightly, the fact remains that, whatever her attitudes, the sister who gives 30 per cent of her time to written exercises spends less time among her staff and hence has less chance of helping their adjustment to her particular ward. We return to examine the ward sister's tasks in a later chapter.

5. The development of attitude surveys

In previous chapters we have described the analysis of certain hospital statistics that throw a little light upon the sickness and wastage of student nurses; and we have referred to the attempts that were made by the research team to analyse the work patterns of the ward sisters. It was, of course, soon apparent that the recording and analysis of the observable behaviour of ward staffs gave only part of the picture; what the girls felt and believed were no less important than what they could, from time to time, be observed to do. We describe in the following chapters some of the methods used to record feelings and attitudes; and we discuss some of the results they produced. It has been suggested to us that we might have given inordinate attention to the analysis of these intangibles; we may be allowed, perhaps, to observe that, less than a century ago, the practice of medicine was transformed by the recognition of what was then invisible even to the sharpest eye, namely, the germ. A study of human feelings in the context of medical practice may, in due course, produce changes no less impressive.

A search for staffing standards

Our first hospital study, at a level deeper than statistical sampling, was undertaken at the invitation of the management committee of a medium-sized hospital, and began as an attempt to understand the problems of staffing its wards. The hospital was known to have a student nurse wastage rate well above the national average, and the problem of providing adequate nursing staff had long been a matter for concern to the lay and nursing administration. It was, all the same, of interest that, although ward staffing ratios already sanctioned by the authorities could not be maintained, the committee perceived their main problem as that of establishing what the 'proper' staffing ratios ought to be. No doubt the clear specification of a target is an aid to reaching it, but at the present state of our knowledge of ward practice it is a forlorn desire to seek for optimum standards. Nevertheless, using methods of job analysis and activity sampling, we were able to show that staffing levels varied significantly not only between comparable wards but also from day to day within particular wards. The load of nursing tasks was unequally distributed between the wards, and the range of administrative tasks, substantial in all cases, varied considerably between one ward sister and another; there were also marked differences in procedures between otherwise comparable wards, and these demanded differing staff complements if they were to be continuously employed.

It was not difficult to show that the stability of the ward team was threatened by fluctuations in staffing levels and by the constant movement of many junior staff at the demand of their training programmes; it was no more difficult to suggest how these variations could be mitigated, nevertheless, by pre-planning in matron's office, in consultation with the principal tutor, and how method study could have suggested a more logical distribution of the work load throughout the different wards and a reduction of the overall burden of administrative and clerical tasks. It would also have been possible, by agreement between the principal tutor and the ward sisters, to establish standard procedures covering all wards, and yet to retain for those in charge of them a degree of independence and discretion in dealing with the problems peculiar to their own wards.

Although objective studies of this nature might eventually suggest some level of ward staffing that balanced the service offered against the effort expended, they could do little or nothing to illuminate the causes of student nurse wastage; this lay at the roots of the shortage of both untrained and trained staff and, thus, of ward staffing problems. In our observations we had many opportunities of talking to the nursing and other hospital staffs, and were always impressed with the volume of spontaneous and unsolicited expression of their attitudes to other people and to their conditions, both in the hospital as a whole and on the ward in particular; these comments strongly suggested several causes of dissatisfaction, and consequently of failure of many student nurses to adjust themselves to their work and training. Such failure often led to their leaving the hospital rather than to achieving the high purpose which had been their inspiration in the beginning, and we decided that it would be useful to record and classify the expressions of views with which that failure seemed to be associated.

The first attitude survey

The step to making a systematic study of attitudes was both natural and easy; our first sample was representative of the nursing staff at the same hospital. It was chosen in an attempt to discover at first hand the attitudes to their work of all grades of nursing staff in the hospital and, as they perceived them, to the physical and psychological conditions affecting its performance. The objective and disinterested recording of subjective and personal opinions has been developed in industry by psychologists in order to reveal to higher management impressions about the environment and personal factors in work situations likely to affect performance, about how these factors interact with one another and about how they might possibly be changed or modified to produce 'desirable' changes in behaviour. (In our hospital studies we had no thoughts about such manipulation.)

The methods most frequently used in studying the attitudes of employees have consisted in:

(a) questions, apparently admitting of unambiguous replies, put either directly or by means of written questionnaires, about the way employees think, feel and are disposed to respond towards their work conditions; the results are classified under the headings already built into the enquiry; and

(b) non-directive interviews in which the interviewer merely records whatever opinions, feeling and wants relative to the work situation are spontaneously expressed by the employees who volunteer both to attend and to disclose their consciousness.

It is important to remember that all questionnaires, whether verbal or written, must pose specific questions, and that their compilers must assume, perhaps too readily, not only that their questions are relevant but also that they are comprehensive, and that there exist answers to them which can be given explicitly. We preferred to use the non-directive interview; in this the interviewer does not ask questions, except to encourage the interviewee, when necessary, to explain or to amplify something which has already been said spontaneously about a topic. The assumption is made that the points raised spontaneously by the interviewee are for him or her those features of the work situation which, at that particular time, really matter. If large numbers of persons sharing the same experience volunteer similar views about the same aspects of them, it is reasonable to suggest that these particular matters are of some importance to them. A party of tourists who have just spent the night in a flea-ridden hotel are unlikely to open the morning's conversation with the representative of their travel agency by airing their views upon, say, the cultural level of the local museums.

The success of the non-directive interview depends, of course, upon the voluntary cooperation of all grades of staff and upon a guarantee that the information offered is both confidential and anonymous, if so desired. A letter written by the head of the research team to individual members of the senior and junior nursing staffs explained the general purpose of the study, and invited the recipient to talk in confidence and anonymity to the team about any hospital and nursing matter which seemed to him or her important, interesting or a substantial source of difficulty or satisfaction. This letter also gave the names of the interviewers, who were already known to many of the staff by sight, from informal conversations in the dining rooms and social contacts in the lounges; it also explained that, on the initiative of the staff, appointments could be arranged with a resident member of the team.

It must, however, be recognized that, in spite of these preparations, this first survey could hardly pretend to be as comprehensive and unbiased as others undertaken later in the research programme, since it followed studies made throughout the hospital into questions of ward staffing. It was already known to all the nurses who attended the interviews that the team was particularly interested in questions of training and recruitment, and for this reason the remarks volunteered tended to keep closely to these matters. For all that, the picture of the nurse's life and problems obtained by interviewing nearly 70 members of the staff, from the matron to the first year student nurses, seems both clear and intelligible; it certainly suggests in what directions there is room for administrative improvement. The results of these interviews, which lasted on average about half an hour and which raised on average about six main points of interest, have been classified by the subjects introduced, and not by any scheme imposed by the research team as representing issues considered by them to be relevant. They are described in the next paragraphs, which are not in any order of importance, measured, for example, by the number of comments passed under any particular heading. In the next chapter, however, we touch upon the validity of quantitative estimates of opinions and attitudes as indicators of problems calling for attention.

Nurses' attitude towards pay

The matron and a senior sister volunteered the opinion that the pay of student and trained nurses was the main source of discouragement to the recruitment and retention of nursing staff. In their view, an allround improvement would solve the problems of student nurse wastage and consequent shortage of trained nursing staff; more people would be recruited and more would complete their training. Another sister suggested that young girls were 'surely under hypnosis when they agreed to accept such a small training allowance. . . . All this business of working for little and setting an example is out of date. . . . Nurses at all levels should be paid according to the responsibility and social value of their work.' (She was not, under the conditions of free interviewing, invited to suggest how these were to be measured.) On the other hand, a junior sister who, as subsequent enquiries showed, had more insight than her seniors, insisted strongly that pay was not the main source of dissatisfaction leading to loss of student nurses. It was, in her view, much less important in the hospital than 'the unfriendly relationships which existed between the senior sisters and their subordinates'.

One or two student nurses feelingly asserted that nursing today was a 'vocation only up to a point'. The rate for the job should be in keeping with the degrees of responsibility involved in it. They did not see why conditions of pay should not be as good as they were in industry. 'What gets us down', said one girl, who claimed to be speaking for her colleagues, 'is that we cannot buy the things our friends in other jobs have.' It was to them unjust, when the pay was so low, that they should be asked, as they frequently were, to work overtime without compensation either in extra off-duty time or in money.

On the other hand, just as many student nurses said that they had no complaint to make about their pay: 'We knew when we came in that the pay would be low.' More than half did not mention the question of pay at all, whether to express dissatisfaction or not. One had to remember that an expensive training was being given and that when in residence the students had amenities such as separate bedrooms and attendance that they might not get at home. Dissatisfaction with pay should not, in our view, be regarded as one of the main reasons why so many student nurses left before completing their training.

35

Food and residence

The food served in the sisters' and student nurses' dining rooms gave little cause for complaint. This happy state of affairs had followed a recent kitchen reorganization; several student nurses thought that meals were 'better than they used to be'. But it was still said that good food was sometimes 'spoiled in the cooking'; the persisting bad feature, however, was the slowness of the service of meals, especially at lunch time, which, in their view, left nurses with little or no time to relax before returning to duty. The second tea served to nurses on night-duty was described as 'terrible'. (The interviewers who had on occasion joined the nurses in this meal agreed.)

The comments made by sisters and staff nurses were somewhat general in nature. Some thought 'that student nurses today probably did not have very much fun as residents', and that perhaps the rather dull social life of the nurses' home explained why some of them withdrew from training. (We did not seek objectively to establish what these women, some no longer young, meant by 'very much fun', but there was, at least on a verbal level, nothing to suggest that, in these affairs, standards vary much from one generation to another.) The living accommodation and conditions provided by many other hospitals for nurses in training was, in the view of the senior staff, 'shocking' and 'it was not to be wondered at that student nurses left in large numbers'. More specific criticisms were made by students in residence. The physical conditions in the home were poor; the building itself was old and 'overrun by cockroaches'; it was situated on a main road and, consequently, very noisy. 'Promises of improvement had often been given but nothing had been done.' It was said by one or two that student nurses had left the hospital because of this. Was it not reasonable to believe that the hospital would attract more nurses and keep them longer if the living conditions of residents were improved? Would it not be possible to estimate the cost of losing nurses and set this off against the cost of improving the home?

But, to the majority of resident nurses, physical conditions were less important sources of dissatisfaction than the unsympathetic and domineering nature of the supervision exercised by the home sisters. The resident student nurses described themselves as not being 'treated in the home like responsible adult people'. 'We are expected to assume heavy responsibilities on duty; in the home we are credited with neither common sense nor self-respect.' The administrative and nursing staff were seen as altogether too old-fashioned and restrictive in their attitude to young people. The home sisters, in particular, 'seemed to have a grudge against human beings in general'. It is true that young girls away from home need to be looked after, that the hospital is *in loco parentis*, and that the anxieties and pressures of ward life may, from time to time, seek release through activities not regarded as entirely ladylike. It is, however, questionable whether, in their struggles against the Prince of Darkness, the student nurses were much aided by the 'petty and humiliating restrictions' of which so many complained. 'Even the privacy of our bedrooms and lockers is not respected by members of the staff who have master-keys.'

36

Hours and off-duty time

The matron and several of her administrative sisters thought that, although the facts were made clear in a selection interview, student nurses on entry did not realize that, in addition to their ward duties, much free time would have to be devoted to study and that this would inevitably restrict their social activities. The hours of work, at that time a minimum of 48 per week, were too many for such an exacting job as nursing; they have since been reduced. The existing split duty system made it difficult for the student nurses to meet friends who, unlike themselves, were free at week-ends. Some nurses said that, in any case, they were too tired to do anything but spend their off-duty time resting in bed.

The matron said she was planning a shift system to improve on the split duties. Senior and junior sisters believed that a workable shift system would both act as a stimulus to recruitment, and help to retain those student nurses already on the hospital books. In their view, however, the matron's scheme would never work, for she had 'not consulted any of the sisters, neither those who had had experience of working a shift system, nor even the sisters on whose wards a pilot study was to be attempted'. . . . The senior sisters had prejudged the issue; 'there would be chaos'. . . . The team were aware that well-intentioned efforts were made to plan off-duty times fair to everyone involved, but it was difficult, with the traditions of seniority long accepted at the hospital, to give student nurses time off at the week-end. It was possible that dissatisfaction with off-duty time was a direct source of student nurse wastage, but it might also have been a manifestation of resentment against the senior staff, who were thought generally to be shown favour in these inflammatory matters. Similar opinions were expressed by staff nurses, but they did not see any valid reason why time off at the week-ends should not be given to all grades of nursing staff in turn, and not only to sisters. Staff nurses sympathized with students, who were apparently expected to be 'married to the profession'; it was accepted that 'they were forced to cancel dates with sweethearts or other promising friends'. The loss felt by the girls was not just that of a particular date foregone; they sensed the loss of goodwill involved in breaking appointments. The student nurses themselves were particularly unhappy that the off-duty roster was often changed 'at the last minute without warning', that it was not published long enough in advance 'to enable student nurses satisfactorily to arrange their private lives', and that 'sisters monopolized all the Saturdays and Sundays'. Off-duty time should, in their view, be allocated so that such inconveniences as being deprived of the company of one's boy friend 'for a whole fortnight' might be avoided. The introduction of a shift system, already the subject of hospital rumour, was heralded as a possible solution to some of these problems.

Student nurses had few complaints to make about the actual number of hours worked, although for one male student the working day was 'tiring even for a man in training'; for one girl student it was 'fatiguing but just sufferable'.

Night duty

Night duty, in the opinion of the matron, involved 'problems of adjustment which were too difficult for some student nurses'; this, in her view, played an inevitable part in wastage. The spell of night duty naturally engendered fatigue which was not dispelled by rest during the day, and eventually created 'a feeling of being everlastingly tired'. It did not occur to the matron that it might be a duty of the hospital to help the student nurses to solve these 'problems of adjustment'. (It was frequently argued that, as in the so-called process of natural selection that lies behind the course of evolution, the progress of the individual nurse should constantly be checked by severe challenges. Only those girls able to overcome them by their own efforts were fitted, in the view of many matrons and tutors, to qualify as nurses. The very great differences in wastage rates between hospitals seems to destroy this argument; if care is taken over the girl's emotional adjustment she will probably survive the most exacting clinical ordeal.)

Some sisters and staff nurses said that students were put on night duty too soon after leaving the PTS. Night duty, in their view, could be very frightening for young girls who had little or no experience on day duty of dealing with patients. Some were said to be terrified of being left alone, particularly on acute medical wards. Emergencies could not always be foreseen by sister; she could not always warn her charges of what to expect nor could she always be present when the unexpected happened. Some girls were reassured when told they could contact sister by telephone should an emergency develop. Unfortunately, some sisters were seen as discouraging the use of the telephone for this purpose. Some students 'were known to have given up nursing as a result of their first spell of night duty'; 'They were afraid of sister.' They knew that if they made a mistake 'they would get no sympathetic consideration'. Other sisters, however, did not think that young nurses discontinued their training because of night duty, although 'some students are capable of dealing with any emergency right from the start and others are just stupidly helpless'. 'A girl who could not quickly adjust herself to night duty would never become a good nurse and, therefore, would not be a loss to the profession if she did leave. The sooner she ceased to be an embarrassment the better.'

Night duty was not mentioned as a problem by all student nurses. On the contrary, several observed that it provided them with welcome opportunities of accepting greater responsibilities and 'acquiring wider experience than was possible on day duty'. There was 'a more friendly atmosphere on nights, and it was possible to learn a lot especially if you had a helpful senior in charge'. Nevertheless, some students had not liked their first spell of night duty, and spoke of it with unconcealed dissatisfaction; some recalled by name friends who had left the hospital for this reason. Other students stated emphatically their belief that they were given unreasonable responsibility when they first went on night duty; their experience on day duty had not prepared them for it; they were not given any helpful instruction. They had 'in theory, only to ask if they didn't know, but in fact *they* were unapproachable; one could not ask *them* anything'. The fear of making a mistake and of 'letting the patient down' was said to be perpetually with them, and was not relieved by the belief that if a nurse did make a mistake she would get no sympathy from the sister. Other disadvantages of night duty said to be experienced by student nurses were the difficulty of study, particularly when preparing for examinations, and the further restrictions placed upon social and recreational activities; 'school friends and boy friends were virtually lost'. Moreover, the spell of night duty was said sometimes to be extended beyond the official duration of twelve weeks. One student had served eighteen weeks, another twenty-two weeks; a third had apparently established a record spell of seven months. She said, 'I dared not complain, or I'd have got more of it; some matrons have no feelings'.

Training

The matron and members of her administrative staff saw some weakness in the current system of training; 'it was too intensive and led to mental indigestion'. They believed that some students who began their training with enthusiasm were later proved to be intellectually incapable of absorbing 'the theoretical aspects of the syllabus', and to be unsuitable for general training. Other students were said to be reluctant about facing the demands which study made upon their leisure time. Liaison between the tutorial and ward staffs was said by the staff of the training school to be poor; practical instruction was not given on the wards, nor were the students brought into contact with the patients when being taught something of the diagnosis and treatment of ailments. (This seemed to be a schism not beyond the power of the Hospital Management Committee to bridge, but nothing systematic was ever attempted.)

Preliminary training school to ward

Sisters and staff nurses knew that their methods were not always those given in the school; what was demonstrated in the school could not, it was said, always be performed on the ward. For example, in the training school three nurses cooperated in doing dressings; three nurses were never available on the ward. Some wards were less well equipped than the training school, where 'there were altogether too many frills'. Nevertheless, it was asserted with confidence that girls who really wanted to be nurses would not find such difficulties insurmountable, although when the senior staff themselves began to dwell upon the obstructions to training, they perceived the need for closer cooperation between tutors and ward sisters. 'Dealing with dummies in PTS was very different from dealing with sick people in bed on the wards.' 'The methods used by some sisters were obsolete and ought to be discarded.' (In spite of this, tutors, it was said, were not encouraged to visit the wards, nor was the Procedures Committee regarded as a particularly effective instrument.)

The communication difficulties perceived by the sisters and staff nurses were also reported by many student nurses. They observed many differences between what they had been taught in PTS and what the sisters, themselves trained in different hospitals, expected them to do. Much of their preliminary training in practical nursing seemed to them 'a waste of time' ... 'a dead loss' since the methods taught differed so much from those in use on the ward. One feels, however, that poor relations exaggerated the problems of accommodating to these differences. The 'vast amount of theory' presented in the training school and in subsequent 'blocks' also failed to illuminate any significant ward experience. This was confusing to young nurses who felt themselves to be, in general, 'full of enthusiasm at the end of their preliminary training, but soon disillusioned and discouraged by the realities of the ward.' They suggested that there was need for detailed instruction on the ward under supervision of the principal tutor, and generally for a closer link in the students' minds between school theory and ward practice. There were in the present situation so many sources of misunderstanding, discouragement and disillusion to young nurses that, in the simple words of one sister about to leave to get married, 'it was difficult to understand why any of them put up with it'.

Introduction to the ward

'The realities of nursing sick people on the ward shocked many young girls.' This was the opinion of several sisters and staff nurses. They also perceived some students arriving in the ward from the training school with the idea that 'they were going to have a nice time' and with a completely unrealistic impression of their new life, derived from films, radio, television and propaganda literature on nursing, including the brochure issued by the hospital. The senior staff felt that the school 'did nothing to dispel this over-glamourized picture'. Some girls were considered too young and naïve when they came on the ward. .... 'They were emotionally off the beam.' Our own observations had shown us that, in the hurry and excitement of the ward, some sisters were sometimes impatient of the inexperience and blunders of their young charges. Probably some of these very blunders stemmed from 'fear of the sister who would give them no consideration if they made a mistake'. The induction of the student into ward work at all levels, psychological, social and clinical, would, in our view, adequately repay detailed consideration and sympathetic experiment. If, for example, she could be given practical experience on the ward while still under the interested and discriminating tutelage of the training school, 'she would not be such a drag upon the sisters', as she now was said to be.

Student nurses were unanimous in volunteering the view that moving from the school to the ward was fraught with difficulties. They perceived their inexperience; they sensed the weight of their responsibilities; they minimized neither. What really shocked and confounded them was that they sensed so little understanding; they felt offered so little help that they gained confidence neither in themselves nor in their seniors. The only sympathy and support they recognized was from their struggling colleagues in the same training school set;

some reported an anxiety to learn, but shrank before the sisters, as an absconding prisoner avoids the alerted sentry. Some sisters were said not to treat their juniors like human beings—'they become emotional and shouted orders which I was expected to understand without explanation, and to carry out without question'. Most students learned very little except caution on their first ward . . . 'somehow, one felt unwanted' . . . 'things were incomprehensible' . . . 'sister had no time to be bothered with you, so you just groped around' . . . 'you just had to stick it and find out all you could; nobody told you anything'. . . . Some students failed to realize how much study they had to do after leaving the training school: five out of ten members of one set were said to have left immediately after going on the ward; they had been seen by the survivors as unable to cope with study on top of their arduous work.

Instruction on the ward

Sisters interpreted the problems of the ward in their own way; some felt that, short of staff, they had little, if any, time to devote to student nurses. The sisters saw themselves as 'battling against death'; they felt obliged themselves to do what was necessary to ensure that it was done not, indeed, quickly and efficiently, but at all. Supervisory and training duties were to them subordinate to such considerations. But, even if they could feel that there was the time, it would still be difficult, in their view, to carry out any systematic instruction because, although student nurses were supposed to remain on a ward for three months, they were, in fact, subjected to frequent and unexpected postings. Most sisters professed not to know why such changes were necessary; they were only aware of conditions making it impossible 'to develop any team spirit on the ward'. (As previously mentioned, some girls stayed, or said they stayed, on night duty for months together.)

Similar views about the difficulties of ward instruction were expressed by staff nurses; they agreed that student nurses were not always shown how to perform unfamiliar tasks on the ward, and that the jobs they were given to do were often far from interesting. The work of absent orderlies or cleaners, for example, necessarily fell upon the junior nurses. There was on some wards a concealed hostility between the senior and junior sisters, so that 'the student nurses were left in a fog'; it was not surprising that they often behaved as if they had no idea of what was happening on the ward. In the view of the staff nurses, the senior sister could find time, were she really so inclined, to instruct the students in her own peculiar methods; she could at least call her staff together for at least ten minutes every day to give them a report, both useful and instructive, on the diagnosis, treatment and progress of the patients. This kind of conference could be expected to arouse the students' interest and, most important of all, give them the experience of active participation in deciding upon the work of the ward.

According to student nurses themselves, the sisters generally did not give them very much helpful instruction on the ward. Some sisters spent too much time 'drinking tea in the duty room, not infrequently waited upon by a student nurse'. The majority of sisters in the hospital did not seem to be interested in teaching their juniors, and were said to discourage questions. One sister replied to the query of a student in search of knowledge, 'Don't you dare to ask me; you should have learned that in the PTS'. There was 'a state of indecision among student nurses' because sisters were 'unapproachable and uncommunicative', particularly about the patients' conditions and treatment. 'You don't have the same interest if you don't know what is wrong', and 'You are more likely to make a mistake if you don't know the reason for the patient's treatment' are remarks which indicate the needs of student nurses. Some sisters thought that 'making casual remarks to student nurses' or 'just ordering them to do things' were adequate vehicles of clinical instruction. A few minutes before a student had attended for interview, the sister had said to her, 'Don't let him (the patient) sit up', but why the patient should not be allowed to sit up was not explained; the student was quite unable to offer any satisfaction to the protesting patient. Some sisters were seen as unable to give orders with ordinary civility. One student, fresh from the training school had been told, 'Go and clean the sluice'; she did not know where the sluice was, nor where to find the gear and materials with which to clean it. One or two sisters 'literally screamed their orders at the nurses'; they were felt never to show the nurses how to do anything and rarely to give them help when they, in their ignorance, made mistakes. A few of the students thought that all hospital staff senior to them tended to regard student nurses as 'skivvies' and to impose upon them as many as possible of the menial tasks of the ward, deliberately depriving them of any chance of helping the patients and of getting real nursing experience.

Interpersonal relations

These interviews soon taught the team that the basic problems of the ward were bound up with simple human relationships in the very special conditions of anxiety, uncertainty and authority common to most hospitals, and we close this chapter with one or two examples of what the interviews revealed of these complex and often distressing emotional conflicts.

Some sisters gave the impression they had often had to deal with student nurses who were not really interested in the patients, 'especially if there was a doctor around'. The students displayed to the sisters 'a glamourized and romantic view of nursing', but were sadly let down when they discovered the illusory nature of both the glamour and romance; as the sisters remarked 'There wasn't a doctor for every nurse'. Sisters met with 'sheer stupidity amongst nurses and lost their patience and sometimes their temper'. Part of the trouble was that 'young people of today had had too soft an upbringing; they were in need of more severe discipline.' One or two older sisters seemed to have developed an austere outlook on life in general, and unfriendly attitudes towards young people in particular; they were seen as the authors, in that hospital, of many of the student nurses' problems. Nor were all of the younger sisters always more sympathetic; the censorious among them had been promoted when 'too young and inexperienced';

some admitted to discouraging the students from asking questions and 'to putting up a bluff to hide their own ignorance'.

Student nurses in turn expressed dread about having to work on certain wards because of the 'domineering and hostile attitudes' of the sisters. In the opinion of the team, such attitudes, more than any other factor, were responsible for wastage, particularly in the first year. Several potentially suitable girls were seen by their friends as having been 'driven out of the profession' by sisters who had subjected them to petty persecutions, who had reprimanded them in the presence of the patients and who had denied them privileges which had been granted to others. 'If a sister got her knife into a student the life of the nurse became a misery.' The students felt defenceless against the criticism of a hostile sister; 'one just has to put up with it or leave the hospital'. One student interviewed had left her first hospital 'because of the domineering attitude of a ward sister'; she had returned to nursing because she liked it, and was now determined to complete her training in spite of all the difficulties encountered on her second attempt. Several student nurses suggested that the attitudes of their sisters had changed for the better since the research team had spent time on the wards, but this may have been no more than a friendly response to what was, for all of them, a singular experience—an opportunity to say what they pleased to a group of persons who seemed, in some respects, to enjoy the status of both matron and doctors.

We must repeat that this was a hospital with a serious staff wastage problem. The attitudes here recorded suggest little but unrelieved difficulties; in fact, when the same hospital was visited several years later its general tone had greatly improved, although the shortage of nurses was still acute. Nor is the hospital typical. The sisters, for example, at another now being studied by the team speak with unanimous affection of their matron; the staff as a whole are secure and their criticism is constructive. Following the attitude study, but without specific advice from the team, a number of improvements in the hospital organization have come about almost spontaneously; an already healthy organism is capable of perceiving and correcting its own faults if the opportunity arises. At other hospitals the team has been deeply impressed with the cheerfulness and resource with which all grades of staff have put up with and even conquered difficulties of accommodation that first became subjects of justifiable complaint during the first World War. If any testimonial to the staff of British hospitals were needed it could be found, like the memorial to Sir Christopher Wren, in the buildings by which they were enveloped.

6. Living and learning

The attitude survey described in the previous chapter arose, and was known throughout the hospital to have arisen, out of a search for the staffing levels thought to be desirable on its wards. This probably led the persons interviewed to offer an undue amount of comment upon this particular feature of hospital life. Those who conducted the survey, nevertheless, were impressed by the comment that was also volunteered upon other hospital affairs; they saw such surveys as instruments for studying the perceptions of hospital staffs as a whole. Since in the early studies of nurse wastage it had begun to appear that the adjustment of the student to her new way of life, including the development of her attitudes towards the patient, was significantly conditioned by her relations to others in the hospital, we felt that these surveys might possibly be developed as a means of determining what these relations might be and upon what they depended.

Our argument was as follows: both student nurse and patient are faced with considerable tasks of adjustment, the student nurse to a way of life, the patient to the path of recovery. It may strike some as novel to suggest that patient care is, for nurse and patient alike, essentially a learning process, something normally thought of in the remote and sheltered confines of a school classroom. But if a patient does not want to recover he can stop himself from doing so; the patient who is worried about domestic troubles cannot give his attention to getting better; with sufficient tutelage any of us can learn to be ill, and some family circles are full of sympathy and encouragement for the potential hypochondriac. Confidence in one's doctor is merely the self-understanding that he engenders, and those who are afraid or who do not wish to understand themselves spend their lives seeking the impossible, namely, the doctor who 'understands' them. We have already suggested that student nurses who, whether through infelicitous teaching or unconscious neglect, have difficulty in learning their tasks, show signs of undue stress and are frequently absent sick; ward sisters learn to adjust more readily to some hospitals than to others. But learning processes, at any level in this life, are more than obedience, however disciplined, however submissive, however unqualified, to instructions, however clear, however appropriate, however authoritative. Patients who feel what may seem an irrational desire to sit up in bed are not helped to adjust themselves to recovery by a peremptory instruction to lie still; nurses who are curious to know why there are marked differences between the procedures used on different wards lose confidence in themselves as well as in their seniors when explanations, even if not strictly logical, are refused. No learning, no adjustment, no progress occurs; there is merely an increase of anxiety, perhaps of frustration, in both nurse and patient alike. A fresh level of understanding is attained only when the subject can rearrange, in the light of the new situation, what is already intelligible and therefore useful. One important element in this process is the opportunity to ask questions that will clear up doubts; since these doubts may be imperfectly known to the learner, they cannot be revealed even to himself, let alone to the teacher, without cross questioning, and this can sometimes threaten to become both unsympathetic and humiliating. Learning occurs most effectively when the doubts in the mind of the learner can be spontaneously voiced when they are to him most insistent. If the learner cannot ask questions or seek clarification when he stands in need of it, his learning process will be retarded, since new knowledge is most easily absorbed when there is an eagerness to use it. The difference between giving learners the opportunity to ask questions, on the one hand, and of denying these opportunities, on the other, is not merely the difference between making learning pleasant or making it laborious; it is the difference between learning and not learning. It is partly for this reason that popular attention is now focused upon the doctor—patient relationship; doctors who withhold information or deny patients the opportunity to ask questions are not merely both making patients feel unsure of themselves and obscuring their own view of the patients' troubles; they are also actively impeding the learning processes that carry them towards recovery. In the same way, the student nurse who feels she is discouraged from seeking clarification of her instructions may sense that this opposes her adjustment to her new life, and, unable to voice her confusion, she may well protest by withdrawing from the hospital. It is not the humiliation of public rebuke for her mistakes but the denial of intelligibility in her work that she so keenly feels, just as to the patient the real enemy is not physical pain but mental anxiety.

This may seem a subjective argument. We nevertheless felt that it would be worth testing. To do so would demand a method of measuring the extent to which those on the wards felt themselves free to ask questions about whatever they liked, or otherwise to communicate with those from whom they might be expected to learn. But before we could devise methods of measuring this perceived freedom of approach, we felt it necessary to classify hospital attitudes without disclosing that our primary interest was in the transparency of communication, particularly in situations of doubt. By conducting general attitude surveys we felt that we might detect specific opinions, beliefs, or prejudices that could eventually form the elements of a statistically significant enquiry. Our first task, therefore, was to gain experience in recording the flow of confidential opinions; in doing so over the course of three years, we have conducted general attitude surveys in six large general hospitals, and, parallel with these, specific studies of cadet schemes, ward sisters' opinions or aspects of organization in another 50 or so. We can refer here to but a small fraction of our total results, and we have chosen to present these in a way that, we believe, illustrates our general thesis, namely, that since the hospital is, and must be by the nature of its task, an institution highly charged with anxiety, among the medical staff, among the senior nurses, among the students no less than among the patients, the outstanding social need of the hospital is the relief of anxiety. This demands enlightenment, understanding, significance, interpretation, meaning, intelligibility: all these depend upon the communication of what is relevant and this in turn depends upon human attitudes. We have tried, from the results of our surveys, to estimate what these may be and how far they differ between hospitals; we did not, of course, at any time try to influence either the views expressed or the choice of subjects about which they were volunteered. We admit that a limitation of the method is that stress tends to be laid on matters about which the staff, being no more than human, want action to be taken rather than upon those with which they are satisfied. We acknowledge this tendency towards painting a picture darker than the scene with a quotation from one of our own reports to a Hospital Management Committee:

> Finally as has been previously indicated, a number of nursing staff felt that this hospital 'was a happy hospital with a wide variety of patients'. 'Conditions have improved tremendously.' 'Pleased to have come into general nursing ... this is a very enjoyable hospital.' The great volume of unfavourable comments which are brought up in this type of survey are specific in nature—that is, they are not representative of an unfavourable attitude to the hospital as a whole. Many of those interviewed, if asked whether they enjoyed working at the hospital, would have replied in the affirmative.

Before briefly presenting our results we may say that, in every hospital, its interpersonal relations, measured by the number of comments spontaneously made by the staff about those with whom they lived and worked, occupied a place in the consciousness of those we interviewed more prominent than that of any other subject. Granted the importance of those relationships, therefore, our next task was to examine their nature.

Summary of results

Table 6.1 gives a classification of the comments, not distinguishing between favourable and critical, passed by the staffs of three of the general hospitals examined. These comments are classified according to the classes of staff who passed them, and the subjects about which they were volunteered.

In deciding upon the size of sample of staff to be invited for interview, the team aimed to see about one quarter of the resident medical staff, the whole of the administrative nursing staff, including the principal tutors, a third of the ward and departmental sisters, a quarter of the trained nurses, a fifth of the junior nurses and hospital cadets, a seventh of the ward orderlies, a tenth of the professional and technical staffs from the laboratories and X-ray departments, and about one-twentieth of the domestic, maintenance, catering and similar staff. Individuals were invited, within these classes, at random; of over a thousand persons invited (some in hospitals other than those here described) only two or three declined to come, and these were all domestic and allied staff. Many more than this in other

Table 6.1

Numbers of comments volunteered by different classes of staff, and by type of comment, for three acute general hospitals—(a), (b), and (c).

(a) *Hospital Q*

Staff category	M.	A.N.	T.N.	U.N.	O.	P.T.A.	A.	Total
Number interviewed	0	17	83	36	12	28	26	202
Topics	Number of comments							
Physical conditions	0	13	64	59	20	33	28	217
Hours of work	0	18	74	78	6	11	18	205
Staffing and methods	0	17	87	19	13	18	23	177
Canteen and food	0	6	68	47	10	21	2	154
Supplies and equipment	0	5	49	20	11	7	21	113
Transport	0	0	0	0	0	0	0	0
Pay	0	2	3	3	8	1	0	17
Interpersonal relations	0	20	257	110	10	120	23	540
Recruitment	0	0	0	0	0	0	0	0
Training	0	8	74	81	16	2	2	183
Social and recreational	0	0	5	5	0	3	1	14
Promotion	0	0	0	0	0	0	0	0
Total	0	89	681	422	94	216	118	1620
No. of comments per interviewee	0	5·2	8·2	11·7	7·8	7·7	4·5	8·0

grades, although not being invited, nevertheless asked if they could be allowed to offer their views; nobody was refused. All who came for interview were given two or three days' notice, were assured that what they might have to say was private and confidential and were invited to bring with them their own list of any matters they might wish to raise, in case they might otherwise forget something. None of these seen objected to the interviewers making written notes of their comments.

The classification of what was said proved a considerable task. It was found that, on average, each person raised about seven topics; their interviews lasted between a quarter of an hour and an hour, with a fairly well marked mode of about half an hour. On the other hand, since the interviews made no attempt to draw their visitors out, except on topics already spontaneously raised, it may well be that between three and ten separate points of interest are the greatest number that most people can carry in their minds as topics to be freely introduced into a conservation, given no outside stimulus that might well tempt them to release more; this influence the team was careful to avoid. However this

Staff category	M.	A.N.	T.N.	U.N.	O.	P.T.A.	A.	Total
Number interviewed	5	13	67	50	22	25	6	188
Topics	*Number of comments*							
Physical conditions	4	6	28	35	13	7	0	93
Hours of work	0	8	57	67	12	18	5	167
Staffing and methods	2	5	28	15	6	1	0	57
Canteen and food	0	13	57	71	21	16	1	179
Supplies and equipment	0	0	1	8	0	1	0	10
Transport	0	0	12	12	8	1	0	33
Pay	1	2	29	29	15	13	0	89
Interpersonal relations	4	11	144	143	36	67	2	407
Recruitment	1	10	78	28	6	21	5	149
Training	3	17	80	65	18	28	2	213
Social and recreational	0	0	28	34	7	9	1	79
Promotion	2	0	2	0	1	2	1	8
Total	17	72	544	507	143	184	17	1484
No. of comments per interviewee:	3·4	5·5	8·1	10·1	6·5	7·4	2·8	7·9

may be, the comments made by any individual were eventually recorded on one large punched card, and classified according to subject. It is worth repeating here that the subject classification suggested itself; the subjects are those freely introduced by those interviewed and the function of the interviewers is that of passively sorting a set of items whose categories have been decided by the nature of the survey material volunteered.

Interpretation of interview material

Before asking what can be read into Table 6.1, it is desirable to make some general observations. First, the frequency with which a topic is raised is not in any way dependent upon the interviewers, though it might well be influenced by collusion—or even innocent previous conversation—between the members of staff interviewed. The team thought that the extent to which persons were expressing the views of others that they did not personally share was small, since they generally gave the impression of speaking with spontaneous conviction; many of them were emotionally involved in the situations they described and nearly all expressed the hope that something would be done about the matters which they felt important enough to raise.

Staff category	M.	A.N.	T.N.	U.N.	O.	P.T.A.	A.	Total
Number interviewed	8	7	32	37	16	16	13	129
Topics	Number of comments							
Physical conditions	0	0	1	4	5	4	3	17
Hours of work	3	8	34	77	13	11	12	158
Staffing and methods	7	1	14	2	1	2	3	30
Canteen and food	5	5	17	33	16	8	8	92
Supplies and equipment	0	0	3	5	0	0	1	9
Transport	0	0	5	19	2	0	2	28
Pay	5	3	11	14	7	9	9	58
Interpersonal relations	24	15	59	58	31	22	12	221
Recruitment	11	15	29	11	6	34	6	112
Training	3	6	28	41	28	11	5	122
Social and recreational	2	0	5	8	1	1	1	18
Promotion	0	0	4	1	0	0	0	5
Total	60	53	210	273	110	102	62	870
No. of comments per interviewee	7·5	7·6	6·6	7·4	6·9	6·4	4·8	6·7

M.   Medical staff
A.N.   Administrative nursing, including matron and her deputies, principal tutor and others of the same rank
T.N.   Trained nursing staff, including ward sisters and staff nurses
U.N.   Untrained nursing staff, including students and auxiliaries
O.   Ward orderlies, domestics and other helpers
P.T.A. Professional, technical and ancillary staff such as laboratory technicians, radiographers and physiotherapists.
A.   Administrative staff, such as records officers and hospital secretaries.

Secondly, the comments of the subordinate staff are often upon highly specific matters that are quite well known to the hospital administration, such as poor quality accommodation or shortage of supplies. We have not attempted in reporting these to go into detail; there is nothing of general interest in the opinions voiced by hospital staff of their local problems of this kind except to say that, however much comment they may excite, it will still be less than the comment passed on interpersonal relations.

Thirdly, comments of an embarrassing personal character, although few in number, have not been included; nor have other comments which were general or vague, as about nationalization or the influences of the welfare state. It must be emphasized that, in our view, comments included under interpersonal relations describe the not-unchangeable state of a system rather than, on the one hand, the individuals who may attract the comments and, on the other, the profession as a way of life. Some comments are based on misconceptions of which the interviewers were aware, but these have been included as well as those based on fact. Indeed, it is particularly important to know of comments based on misapprehension, so that action can be taken to make the situation more fully understood. Certain comments may appear irrational or destructive; they nevertheless represent a dissatisfaction of the staff, and should not be ignored. There were, of course, many issues raised which were already sensed by the hospital management, but, even so, a record of the extent and nature of the feeling of different groups about them was valuable.

Fourthly, dissatisfaction expressed in all hospitals appears to be centred around a few main areas which can be further reduced into two categories. The first contains staffing, pay, hours, living conditions, training and promotion, complaints about matters which can be dealt with by the appropriate machinery, on either a national or local level. The second category contains the less tangible problems of communications, social relations, and personal security. Here, different treatments are necessary and, as the action required is largely to change individual perception and awareness, it is clearly dependent for success upon long-term policies. Some attention to the tangible factors, however, will be a sound first move, since it will increase the confidence and trust that employees must have in their own hospital management if the psychological climate is to be improved.

Both in Table 6.1 and in the following paragraphs no attempt has been made to place items in order of importance; and it could be argued that this would be impossible. All classes of problem interact and the hospital must be considered as an integrated whole. Nevertheless, the first conclusion to be drawn from Table 6.1 is the preoccupation of the hospital staffs with difficulties of interpersonal relations; these attract, in all hospitals, more comment than any other subject. In making this classification, moreover, we have been careful to include under interpersonal relations only these relations as such. For example, statements that the dispensary is slow to provide drugs or that the diet kitchen tends to confuse the names of the patients are not entered under interpersonal relations, but under supplies and equipment. But a comment that the pharmacist wilfully keeps student nurse runners waiting and so obliges the ward sister to go herself to see about the prescription is entered under interpersonal relations, though it may be strictly no more than the pharmacist innocently emphasizing his own status. Even in Hospital Q, where relations could be described only as bad, and where this is fairly reflected in the great volume of comment, a measurable, if small, percentage was offered in praise of members of the training school, who were thought to do their work bravely in the face of difficulty and even discouragement said to be engendered by others within the hospital. A detailed study of the types of comment so classified suggests frequent failures of communication; these were occasionally understandable in terms of pressure of work or of the removal of the records by forgetful doctors, but were more frequently attributed to the authoritarian traditions that, for a variety of reasons, hospital practice has inherited. Nevertheless, to improve such attitudes does not necessarily demand, as some imagine, a change in human nature itself; Hospital S, for example, which has a significantly low proportion of comments in this field was, five years ago, an unhappy hospital, judged by any standards. A recognition by the management committee of its communication problems, and a sustained effort by a new matron to improve them, achieved striking results. It will, however, be some time before the public reputation of the hospital as attractive to student nurses is restored to its previous high level; recruitment is still a serious problem and the recent improvement of internal morale will need to be sustained for several years before the flow of local recruits is likely to ensure that the hospital will be adequately staffed. There is no reason to believe that this will not eventually occur.

The recruitment problems of Hospitals R and S, which had been associated with the presence of the investigators in the hospitals, are reflected in the volume of comment about this subject. None of the 202 persons interviewed at the other hospital specifically mentioned it; this was not because the other hospital had no recruitment problems whatever, but because these problems had not passed the threshold level at which they begin to form a subject of everyday conversation, much less of anxiety. Recruitment difficulties, for example, invoke explanation in terms of inadequate pay; it is easy to suggest that girls will be attracted to nursing if they are offered higher wages. Very few staff at Hospital Q pass any comment about pay; it is in the two hospitals that are comparatively shorthanded at which this is in the forefront of the consciousness. While 202 staff at Hospital Q pass only 17 remarks about pay, 317 at Hospitals R and S pass as many as 147. It is also interesting to note how little the staffs of all three hospitals refer to promotion; while those outside the service who are familiar with the young industrial careerist may regard this with approval, there are disadvantages in this widespread contentment to stay in a subordinate position. Nursing seems to be one profession in which there is in fact plenty of room at the top; there is a serious shortage of qualified senior staff of all kinds, and many hospitals have long sought in vain not only assistant matrons and principal tutors, but even matrons themselves. We met in the course of our studies several excellent sisters who, if they mentioned promotion at all, did so only to emphasize the satisfactions of continuing to run their own wards.

All hospital staffs had much to say about their hours of work. A glance at the tables shows that it is in this respect that the three hospitals most strongly resemble each other; Hospital Q, that has no chronic shortage of staff, comments just as much upon its hours of work as do Hospitals R and S, from which there is also so much reference to recruitment and to pay. It is a testimonial to the profession that there is little complaint of long hours as such. Most of the comments are about the uncertainties of off-duty time; we could not be sure whether the majority of the observations were well founded, or whether to complain about the duty roster is merely to do one's homage to the mythology of nursing. Many nurses certainly seemed convinced that the ingredients of the change-list and of the short-notice variations made in it go little beyond favouritism and seniority. No subject could form a better focus for starting or improving a system of joint consultation within a hospital than the preparation of duty lists. The views expressed by the staff about such aspects of technical organization of hospitals as staffing duties, methods and procedures or the supply of services and equipment vary greatly from one hospital to another and no general comment seems necessary here; the management committees of Hospitals R and S were well aware of their chronic shortages of nursing staff and had always been generous in the provision of physical resources.

Interpersonal relations

It was in Hospitals Q and R that the problems of communication came out so strongly in the interview programme. The unforgettable impressions gained by the team are of the persistent difficulty of making any meaningful upward contact; most nurses and ward staff at all levels saw themselves encumbered with a hierarchy actively and openly dedicated to frustrating those whose business lay on the wards; even the sisters spoke at times as if their successes with the patients were as much a victory over their superiors as over death itself. It is impossible in a report of this kind, intended to encourage the objective study of hospital problems, to give illustrations from our experiences without creating an unfavourable impression that would all too undeservedly be attached to better hospitals. The opposition these hierarchies aroused among the subordinate staff in some hospitals may perhaps be suggested by a simple catalogue of words used by those interviewed at one of them; all anecdote and incident are omitted: aloof, brainless, degrading, dictatorial, fear, ignorant, inconsiderate, interference, niggling, obstinate, pecking order, petty, regimentation, restrictions, sarcastic, snappiness, spying, tyrannical, unapproachable, uncooperative, unfriendly, unmannerly, unrest. These are, admittedly, words actually used to describe to us the conduct or attitudes (or their consequences) of particular staff grades as perceived by others, but, if we are permitted to interpret our experience, we suggest that they should not simply be so regarded; they are the terms of some timeless dialogue, between those who, on the one hand, share, and, on the other hand, do not share, the immediate stresses of the bedside in certain hospitals. For, as we have observed earlier in this chapter, the hospital is an institution cradled in anxiety: the consultant can never be wholly confident of his diagnosis, even although he declares it to the assenting echoes of his retinue; the sister can never be wholly sure that she will successfully handle the next crisis, even although she has ruled her ward with a rod of iron these 30 years; the patient is worried, not about himself alone, but also about his dependents, even although they are joined in a conspiracy to assure him that by tomorrow he will be his usual self and back among them. In situations of anxiety one seeks two supports: a senior on whom one can rely, and an understanding of what might happen next. There are some who, placed in senior or responsible positions in such a culture, regard it as a weakness even to seek information, much less advice or opinion, from their subordinate; their main concern is that the fortress of their knowledge and experience shall seem invulnerable; a simple device for ensuring this is to close the fortress to inspection. The subordinate is thus never encouraged to ask questions, since questions may test the superior's defences and even allow the sawdust to trickle out. And since, in management as in war, the surest form of defence is to attack, the insecure or inadequate person, carried by circumstances to a commanding height, will be concerned not to allow the enquiring initiative to pass into the hands of the subordinates; he defends himself against the disclosure of his own shortcomings by aggressively canvassing those of others, and by astutely avoiding any engagement that is likely to question his right to be in charge. An administrator who repels his new and eager subordinate as a worrying nuisance soon has the satisfaction of seeing the subordinate become so frustrated as to be incapable of constructive thought. To at least one member of this team, one of the most gratifying trends in modern hospital practice is the willingness of younger doctors to say, in reply to the questions of a layman, 'I am sorry, but I do not know. Can you suggest how we might be able to find out?' It was also impressive to hear the new matron of a large Midland hospital, faced by the starched array of her sisters' meeting, say in reply to a technical question about some procedural circular, 'Well, girls, would you believe it? That makes two of us. Can anybody tell us both the answer?' Such candid self-revelation and such unassuming self-confidence seem still comparatively rare, perhaps because the patient still demands of his doctor an omniscience to which no mortal man can attain; one certainly gains the impression that many doctors, obliged to act such a part for the reassurance of their patients, eventually grow identified with it, like the crow in the fable, flattered by the fox to believe that she had the voice of a nightingale. The same may not seldom be said of matrons; in situations that, to the young nurse, are charged with unconquerable surges of self-reproach, guilt and even remorse, and by suggestions that had one but done something different from what one actually did, the patient might have lived, there is a constant demand for emotional support and for a sharing of meaningful experience. But what if, in these tentative approaches, the senior should be proved wanting, unwilling to answer the questions, unready to remove the doubts, unable to offer conviction to the hesitating junior? In some hospitals, the system of authority, rigid but insecure, must continually strive to protect itself against such undermining challenges and, sooner than admit the weaknesses of its human foundations, will deny the opportunity to call them into question. In the extreme, we find subordinates who, in their perceptions of the hierarchies under whom they serve, can think only in terms of the words used in the catalogue set out earlier in this paragraph. Even in happier organizations the principal defence mechanism of the insecure manager is a refusal to listen to what is said to him, and the vast majority of the human problems of industry are both aggravated for this reason and insoluble until it is corrected. There is now considerable evidence to suggest that, in institutions strongly dependent upon up-to-date information, the superior who displays inflexible or unsympathetic attitudes towards his immediate subordinates has probably first perceived them in his own superior; the matron, for example who is unsure of the support that, in her own anxious moments, she will be accorded by the hospital management committee (even supposing she is allowed to meet it) is likely to develop an unapproachable or even hostile attitude towards her own ward sisters. It has been shown in the course of this study that the ward sister transmits to her staff the attitudes she perceives in her superiors (see Table A5.3, Appendix 5, page 91). It is to the deeper analysis of these human factors that we turn in the next chapter. It was these surveys of hospital opinion which suggested the form which this analysis should take.

7. Attitude and belief as hospital characteristics

(This chapter should be read with close reference to Appendixes 5 and 5a)

These attitude surveys suggest that some student nurses continue to find it difficult to adapt themselves, even after their first year, to life on the ward. The differences between hospitals, however, in the average wastage rates of the student nurses during their early months is so impressive that we should seek better to understand them; in this search the specific comments of the student nurses about their problems may be helpful.

The statistical analysis of the results of the surveys encourages us to search for structure in these difficulties of adjustment. One question in particular seemed to us to be sufficiently important to demand an investigation in depth. Are the difficulties that the student nurses experience likely to derive from what is often regarded as the authoritarian tradition of the nursing profession, long established and permanent, or are they symptoms, characteristic of organizational disorders, perhaps temporary and tractable, at particular hospitals? In other words, is it some incurable preoccupation with rank and seniority latent throughout the profession as a whole, although coming to the surface in particular hospitals, that repels and disheartens all but the toughest of the junior nurses, those likely to survive and to carry forward their cauterizing brand into a new generation? Or are there in these particular hospitals local, and perhaps temporary, failures of morale symptomatic of some internal malfunction? These questions are important: if the difficulties arise from a universal preoccupation with status, the outlook for the profession must be sombre; the likelihood of changing what is said to be the authoritarian outlook of the nursing hierarchy within one generation is remote, even supposing that such changes are necessary or even desirable in themselves. If, on the other hand, the difficulties which the student nurses in certain hospitals have in making friends of their superiors stem from administrative or organizational shortcomings confined to these particular hospitals, it may not be beyond human contrivance to do something about it soon.

To summarize our conclusions before describing our methods and our experimental results we may say that the evidence suggests that the difficulties of the girls derive largely from failures in the organization of the particular hospital, rather than from any supposed rigidity within the profession itself. Indeed, what is often described as its authoritarian tradition, which rarely fails to impress the bedside visitor unused to hospital life, may be a support vital for those within it. Certainly the third year student who may complain about what she imagines to be the privileges of her seniors will be speaking in a different tone three years later, should she herself by then become a junior sister; the facility with which those who climb the ladder of promotion also adopt the outlook of the levels to which they climb is impressive, and suggests to the student of human affairs some self-sustaining professional defence mechanism against the threats and tensions of responsibility. A system of authority seems to be as necessary for the student nurse to accept as it is for the matron and the ward sister to exercise; the question for us is of the spirit with which the system of authority is informed.

Specific questions from general attitudes

Hierarchy or status

When we classify the thousand or so remarks upon personal relations made by nurses of all ranks in the course of these free interviews, we find that they suggest a few simple ideas. Some of these we may try to describe. Consider, for example, the concept of status, that is, of the privileges, respect or authority granted to or demanded by certain persons by reason of their office or seniority alone. We heard a great deal of criticism by the junior nurses of the allocation of hours set out in the off-duty rota; they often felt that their superiors were unfairly given the best night to be out. This could be a source of intense indignation, since girls who had been banking upon a particular evening off often discovered at the last moment that they were to remain on duty. It is only fair to say in defence of most hospitals that on investigation the number of cases of justifiable complaint was much smaller than one would have imagined from the volumes of protest that were voiced, however deep the individual disappointments. Nevertheless, there was a strong belief in particular hospitals that, in preparing the off-duty rota, the only consideration was seniority or rank within the nursing hierarchy. If, therefore, those in senior positions in a given hospital expressed unambiguously the belief that rank was, and should be, the main criterion adopted for allocating desirable hours, we may take it that this particular hospital displayed hierarchical commitment.

In other hospitals, we met senior nurses, including matrons, who, in private conversation, regretted that the nursing staff was so scattered at meal times; we also met the contrary opinion. Some large hospitals had as many as five different dining rooms, each, apparently, designed to ensure that the nursing staffs of different ranks did not mix with each other off the wards. While few would suggest that the profession ought to adopt a principle of one staff-cafeteria, in which the matron, sisters and nurses of all grades queue in the order of their arrival for their meals, we met thoughtful matrons who would have liked to persuade their sisters that less segregation might be observed at meal times. But we also found sisters who openly expressed the view that status concentration at meal times was essential to the efficiency of the hospital, that is, presumably, to the well-being of the patients. If, therefore, at any hospital it were possible to determine how many of the senior staff believed that the nurses of different ranks should not mix during their meals, we would have a further index of the rigidity of its nursing hierarchy.

These two indicators are drawn from the social life of the hospital. But it is also necessary to suggest how far such hierarchical inclinations might affect the learning situation on the ward. We found, for example, that about half the senior staffs of the hospitals whom we interviewed believed that student nurses should be taught in the training school that they must not speak to the doctor unless the doctor spoke first to them. We cannot be sure that this is necessarily evidence of hierarchical commitment because some sisters, for example, might, from direct experience, believe that the doctor's task is difficult enough already without his being distracted by what he might feel to be the chatter of eager teenagers. This belief seems, nevertheless, to be the inheritance of a previous age, when little children were to be seen and not heard. In some hospitals, indeed, the sisters shooed their junior nurses off the wards just before the main medical rounds took place. The sisters who did this no doubt had good reason to recall complaints by doctors that too much ward activity might interfere with the examination of their patients. Hence, although the extent to which sisters believed that their junior nurses should be taught not to approach the doctors might be evidence of their commitment to hierarchical ideas, it was not used for this study. We chose instead the extent to which ward sisters believed that they themselves and only themselves should always deal with the consultants who visited their wards, however many consultants might happen to turn up. This seemed to us to suggest how far the senior nurse on the ward was willing both to allow her junior to get the experience of discussing cases with those from whom she might learn most and to gain a little experience and responsibility, to use, perhaps, on her own initiative should the ward, at some future date, come under pressure and the sister be unable to deal with everything herself. The dyed-in-the-wool authoritarian can always be recognized by her unwillingness to allow any short-circuiting of the official channels, or any sharing of the power vested in herself.

Our fourth indicator of hierarchical attitudes was a measure of the reliance which the ward sisters placed upon their paper work. We had discovered, during our observations of how the ward team spent its time, that some sisters gave about 30 per cent of their day to paper work and activities closely associated with it out of as much as 60 per cent to administration all told; others gave as little as 10 per cent out of 25 per cent respectively. Granted that lives of patients are at risk and that information about their progress and treatment must be accurate; granted that many persons not readily able to meet face to face need to have access to this information. For all this, there is a limit to the authority that should be expected of written records; in the constant change and emergency of the ward one has to admit the responsibility of the human being to observe, to decide and to act irrespective of what might or might not be dictated by the papers. While nobody would advocate for hospital wards the example of Messrs Marks and Spencer, who have, with striking effect, decimated their written records and insisted upon their staffs talking to each other instead, we suggest that the emphasis that the sister places upon paper work is a measure of the extent to which, as a person, she would sooner rely on what is down in black and white than she would upon the richer, if occasionally less reliable, faculties of her own staff. It is again a mark of the true authoritarian to place the responsibility upon the paper system rather than upon the living person; the French, with their ample vocabulary of womanly weakness, actually have a name for her, *la paperassière*.

Hence, by measuring the specific responses of the ward sisters to four particular statements, namely, about the need (a) to give precedence to seniority in settling the off-duty rota; (b) for nursing staffs of the same rank to keep together at meal times; (c) for the ward sister always to deal with the consultants herself; and (d) to prefer the written record, we have been able to construct an index of hierarchical commitment. We found two interesting results. First, this commitment ranges very widely. There are some sisters who display in each of these four areas the most extreme hierarchical conviction; others hold contrary opinions. Secondly, there are very great differences between hospitals in the average commitment of the ward sisters to these hierarchical beliefs. While within any one hospital the beliefs of the individual sisters are widely spread, the average level in one hospital may be significantly higher or lower than the average level in another (see Appendix 6, page 101).

Student nurse integration

We may, in the same way, use our free interview material to define the attitudes of the ward sister towards the integration of the student nurse into her ward team. In measuring hierarchical commitment we have as far as possible tried to keep our specific responses clear of statements to do with instruction or training of the student. But we observed, either in the course of our ward studies or in the recollections of the student nurses, many situations which must have influenced their development profoundly. In the free interviews, for example, many student nurses remarked that their sisters always seemed too busy to spend time on explaining to the student nurse how to do what she had been told to do; Table 4.2 illustrates the very small amount of ward time which some sisters seem able to give to their juniors. The example is not chosen to exaggerate the point; it is typical of the hospital from which it was drawn. There were many sisters, too, who complained of the pressure of work and of the number of matters they were forced to attend to before they could devote time to training. Hence, we set out to measure the attitudes of the sisters on whether or not they felt they could find time to give to the student nurse only after they had disposed of more important matters.

We found, on the other hand, that many student nurses had been regularly brought by their sisters into conferences with the whole ward team. At these conferences not only had the progress and condition of the patients been discussed but so also had the problems of the staff and of the hospital organization. Some student nurses spoke with feeling about the lack of these consultations in their experience, but when we managed to steer our conversations with the sisters towards these points we were frequently told that there was no time to organize such conferences and that, in any case, they were not worth the time they would take up. We do not know much about learning processes in general, whether in hospitals or elsewhere, but there is evidence that all successful training offers to the student nurse the opportunity to ask questions about her present experiences and to discuss her problems with others who are also learning. If we know, therefore, whether or not sisters regard such ward conferences as worthwhile, we have at once an indication of their attitude to training. We therefore specifically measured this attitude among our ward sisters.

Our third indicator of the sister's outlook upon integration and training was the extent to which she believed that it was her responsibility to explain to the student nurse any instructions sent to the ward from her superiors. Here again, we find a wide divergence of perception; there were some who would regard such efforts as a sign of weakness; subordinates who are offered explanations may retaliate by questioning policies. It was sincerely felt by other sisters that there was no time to explain, much less justify, what perfectly competent people had already decided; others equally sincerely believed that, since, in emergency, the nurse had often to act upon instantaneous and arbitrary instructions, she should not be encouraged to be inquisitive about them. This is a real problem; the point of view is honest and well-intentioned, and it is easy for outsiders to misrepresent what lies behind it. Nevertheless, whatever the perception of the ward sister, her conviction that she should not explain 'higher instructions' to the student nurse must not seldom militate against the girl's assimilation to the ward team.

Fourthly, we have chosen as an indication of the ward sister's attitude towards her juniors the extent to which she feels that she can set high standards of work without herself becoming disliked. In an age when many sisters believe that most young people have had too soft an upbringing, that parents do not exercise enough discipline over their children, or that education today is too theoretical, it is easy for them to express the opinion that if they ask high standards of their nurses they will be personally disliked in return. In fact, we found that this last opinion was held by considerably less than half the sisters. It nevertheless appeared to us to be a meaningful indication of the spirit in which the sister set out to engender high standards of performance in the nurses and so was included in our small battery.

We have therefore measured the attitudes of the sisters towards student nurse integration by testing their responses to four specific matters: namely, whether there is time to instruct the nurses amid the pressure of all other ward duties, whether conferences of the ward team are worth the trouble and time that they would take to organize, whether it is necessary to explain instructions coming down from above and whether it is possible for the sister to demand high standards of her nurses without becoming personally disliked by them. Again we find that the measure of this attitude varies widely between sisters and also that its average level in particular hospitals differs widely from its average level in other hospitals. The variation between hospitals, as in the case of hierarchical commitment, is very significantly greater than the differences between individual sisters (see Appendix 6, page 102).

Status and integration not correlated

We find, however, that there is no relation between these two sets of attitudes (see Appendix 6). We find this result whether we take the sisters individually or whether we compare the averages in particular hospitals. (This is a revision of a conclusion expressed in R. W. Revans's paper of 11 January 1961 to the Manchester Statistical Society. In the earlier paper he attributes to the training block certain attitudes of the sister—towards always dealing with the consultants herself; and towards the need for more and more paper work—which are manifestly attitudes to status commitment. If these re-assignments are made the result given here is confirmed.) By saying that there is no relation we mean that sisters who have extremely authoritarian attitudes, that is, sisters who display marked status commitment, may nevertheless have sympathetic attitudes to student-nurse integration and vice versa; we mean also that sisters with little or no hierarchical commitment may nevertheless have unfavourable attitudes to training and vice versa. We also find that a hospital with an average status commitment that suggests institutional rigidity may (or may not) be staffed with sisters whose average attitudes to integration and training are sympathetic and favourable: or that a hospital which has little collective commitment to status may (or may not) display attitudes unfavourable to student integration. This is an interesting result, because it suggests that if the ward sister's attitude to integration is—as our free interviews with the student nurses suggest—significant in determining whether those students will remain to complete their training, we must look elsewhere than to status commitment to discover on what, if anything, that sister's attitude to integration is founded. The observational fact, mentioned above and brought out in Appendix 6, that some effect, specific to a particular hospital, helps to determine the training attitudes of the sisters who serve there means that this search may well be worthwhile.

The sister's perception of her superiors

Our observations on the floor of the ward showed that in most hospitals ward sisters are, from time to time, necessarily under considerable pressure. In saying this we do not suggest that they are, in fact, so busy that they cannot, for long periods together, attend adequately to their work, nor even that those wards which seem most busy cause the greatest anxiety to the staff who work on them. Elsewhere we suggest that a high activity rate may indeed be a sign of high morale and of well-adjusted student nurses; the evidence is that hospitals with a rapid turnover of patients tend to show a low wastage rate among the nursing staff. Many student nurses, too, suggested in free interview that no other satisfaction could compare with being run off one's feet in the interests of the patients; hospital cadets, not yet tarnished by the realities of institutional experience, rated the opportunity to do some useful hard work as the only reward their life had to offer. However this may be, we were also interested in how the sister spends her time and particularly in the attitude which she has towards those who would appear to influence the effectiveness with which she is able to work.

We found from the free interviews with the ward sisters that their outlook on life is strongly coloured by many features of the hospital organization outside their wards, from the speed with which the medical records section deliver information when asked for it, to the cooperativeness of the engineer in mending a chair or putting a new washer on a dripping tap. It was, however, out of the question to sample on a numerical basis the responses of the sisters towards all of these organizational influences and we finally selected for analysis four influences decisive among the sister's multifarious activities.

The first of these is the attitude of the sisters towards the medical staff for whom they work. We have noticed, without trying to make any statistical record of our impressions, that there are many doctors who regard the work of the nurses as something useful but inferior, as a businessman regards the work of his typist or a pilot the ministrations to his passengers of the air hostess. Some sisters speak with emotion in these affairs, and we were given examples of doctors completely ignoring or even ridiculing suggestions made by sisters about the treatment of the patients. ('Lazarus had to fall back on Jesus Christ. *Our* patients have Mr X.' . . . a Lancashire ward sister on consultants.) In this particular analysis, however, we merely measured the extent to which the ward sisters felt that the doctors were accorded—by relatives, patients, and other doctors—too great a share of the credit for any success which the ward team might achieve. We found, for example, that in certain hospitals the ward sisters were practically unanimous in their view that the doctors took too much of this credit; in other hospitals not one sister imputed to the medical staff this exaggeration of their role. As in other attitudes which we have attempted to quantify, there were very great differences between hospitals in this relationship. While the extent to which the doctor assumes the credit for what is achieved may not measure the pressures upon the sister, the most casual observation reveals that it influences the cheerfulness with which she goes about her work. Ward sisters may be a class well-tempered in the flame of experience, and they may often maintain an illusion of detachment. But the outside observer who spends many hours among them very soon recognizes the immense influence that is exercised on them by the doctors; a few words of appreciation or an admission by the doctor that such and such a suggestion from a sister has altered his view of a case often make not only the average sister's day, but, by this analogy, her whole life.

The perception held by the sisters of their matron is hardly less important than their perceptions of the doctors. While, in our view, the exact functions of hospital matrons and in particular their relation to the ward sisters seem to deserve more thought than they are usually given, the matron is the most important individual on the horizons of the sisters. The extent to which she seemed to be in touch with her sisters' problems and, moreover, able to do much about them was a source of voluntary comment by almost every sister; the average level of appreciation implied in this comment differed more widely between hospitals than any other systematically recorded.

We sought in this area to measure what appear to the sister to be two important influences. The first is the extent to which the matron's office seems to be in touch with the problems of the ward; this was mainly judged by the speed and understanding with which the nursing staff on the ward would be reinforced by the matron or her deputy in times of emergency or of particular difficulty; it was also judged by the sympathy with which the matron's office treated special requests from the sisters for equipment or supplies. Although these requests might eventually be turned down, the sisters were normally quick to grasp whether the matron's office understood and supported the recommendation or not. Secondly, we tried to observe the attitude which the ward sisters had towards participation in their regular meetings with the matron and her staff; some sisters spoke of this meeting with enthusiasm, saying that it did more to strengthen the link between the matron and her lieutenants than any other device in the hospital calendar. Other sisters were less enthusiastic; an outside observer soon notices great differences between these meetings in different hospitals; some which are conducted with little comment from the sisters' side may break up with a release of tension that is illuminating. In particular, the sisters judge the effect of the matron's meeting upon the running of their wards by the extent to which suggestions put forward at the meeting are eventually acted upon; nothing is apparently so frustrating as to spend a great deal of time discussing some particular problem at the matron's meeting and discover in the course of time that nothing can be done about it. We therefore chose, as an estimate of her confidence in her superiors, the extent to which the sister perceives these discussions as producing positive results.

Our fourth factor aimed at assessing the sisters' estimate of her superiors was the extent to which she believed that the ancillary departments of the hospital such as the dispensary, the diet kitchen, the pathological laboratory, the X-ray department and so forth, appeared to recognize that they existed primarily to help the wards. However uncharitable it may be to suggest that some ancillary departments are unmindful of this, the fact remains that we heard many dark allusions to those who suited their own convenience. The growth of functional specialism in any organization, whether a hospital, a town hall or a coal-mine, always brings with it a concentration of technical expertise that may threaten to divide the experts from those who need their services; this tendency to isolation is likely to become worse if the technical specialist feels that his skill may be threatened by still newer forms of professional innovation. We found, for example, that some dispensers felt the growth of ready-made drugs or tablets was a threat to their technical skill and this, according to the sisters, made them at times difficult to handle. In other hospitals the specialist departments complained that they were unable promptly to attend to the demands of the wards because these were ill-formulated. We therefore invited all the sisters to reveal their attitude to the cooperativeness of other departments; evidently, if a ward sister is under pressure and in need of information or help from some other department of the hospital, it can only add to her apparent difficulties if, in her opinion, this other department seems unaware that its central function is to help the patients and those who look after them.

We have in this way measured the attitudes of the sisters towards the effectiveness of the help given to them by their superiors, or towards the general functioning of the hospital organization as it is motivated or controlled by those superiors. We find that the average scores of the sisters differ very greatly indeed between one hospital and another, more so than do the averages of the scores suggesting either attitudes towards hierarchy or status, or attitudes towards the integration and training of the student nurses (see Appendix 6, page 102). This is perhaps no very surprising result: the ward sister who is under pressure will be correspondingly conscious of the extent to which her superiors are, in fact, able to help her. Since there are, even to the most casual observer, differences between the organizational effectiveness of otherwise comparable institutions, it is easy to believe that these differences will be noted and responded to by the ward sisters. But the second major conclusion is more interesting: attitudes of sisters towards nurse integration, although not correlated with their attitudes towards hierarchy or status commitments, are very significantly correlated with their perception of their superiors and of the organization that their superiors control. This suggests that, insofar as the student nurses are in fact influenced by the treatment they get from their ward sisters, and particularly, insofar as this treatment helps to determine their wastage from the training courses, it is to the relations between the sisters and their superiors in particular hospitals that we should give our attention; attitudes towards hierarchy and seniority as such do not seem to influence the sister's outlook on these matters. The problem is not therefore to change an entire professional culture; it is to alter the attitudes of the senior staff in particular hospitals. Until we know a great deal more about the influences which form these attitudes it is unlikely that much progress will be made in this direction. For all that, the task is not impossible; the differences between otherwise comparable hospitals are so great that their causes might well be observable, and when causes are known remedies can perhaps be found.

8. The hospital as a unity

The evidence of the previous seven chapters leads towards one conclusion: there are in any hospital several characteristics, shared by all who work or are treated there, which can be measured and which, when measured, suggest that every hospital may differ significantly in these characteristics from other hospitals. There is a characteristic stability of staff, particularly of ward staff; there is a mean length of stay of patients in particular diagnostic groups characteristic of the individual hospital; at the end of chapter 4 we suggest that these two factors, of staff stability and of mean length of stay are, in large samples of comparable hospitals, significantly related. Our attempts to measure the attitudes of ward sisters towards their superiors and towards their subordinates suggest that these are also related, but that neither follows the patterns of the sisters' attitudes towards hierarchy, status or professional precedence as a determinant of hospital morale or behaviour. We may now ask, as it was suggested in the study of the patients' attitudes by Anne McGhee (see chapter 4), whether 'the atmosphere of the ward' is likely to be related to the recovery rate of the patients. Does the common characteristic that seems, in the sample of five Lancashire hospitals, to enter into both staff stability and patient recovery, also help to determine the 'atmosphere of the ward', or, to turn the question inside out, is there any relation between duration of patient stay and staff stability, on the one hand, and the 'atmosphere of the ward' (whatever that may be), on the other?

Medical and surgical patient stay

To test this hypothesis, we collected statistics, and interviewed several hundred ward sisters, at 15 acute or mainly acute general hospitals in the Midlands and North of England; all except one were in the Manchester or Sheffield Regions, the other in the Leeds Region; none were teaching hospitals. One of the research team spent over a year in visiting these 15 hospitals to collect statistics of mean length of patient stay and of staff wastage, and although those familiar with hospital records may ask whether he could possibly have obtained any figures of value by doing so, we can only answer that we believe he did. The research worker concerned was a recently retired Director of Education, a physicist by early training, and a man who had spent a lifetime dealing with both professional men and bureaucrats, as well as the records with which they work. He collected, from the monthly reports to the Hospital Management Committees, the numbers of patients discharged in certain diagnostic groups common to all the hospitals, much as described in chapter 3, and by weighting for numbers of patients, established two grand hospital average lengths of stay, one for all general medical, the other for all general surgical cases; these two parameters we call here M and S. Once the diagnostic groups had selected themselves, the task, although tedious, was not difficult. The essential quality of the research worker was not his understanding of statistics or of sampling methods, but his ability, acquired from a lifetime of experience in a London town hall, to interest the consultants, as well as the assistant records officers, in what he was trying to do. Much preparatory social research, whatever the purists have to say, can be started only if existing statistical material is used; if much of this is imperfect it is the business of the research worker to identify the character, and to allow for the magnitude, of its imperfections, and this he can do if he has the ability to work with the clerks who prepare the records. The need is imperative enough almost to merit the identification of a new branch of research: as theology is supported by the discipline of interpreting scriptural texts, namely, exegesis, so the student of society needs the support of those skilled in reading and verifying the records kept by clerks at the places to which they refer, and under the pressures and distractions of daily life.

Stability of qualified ward staff

The stability of the ward staff was not easy to estimate. We were soon obliged to study qualified staff only, namely, ward sisters, junior sisters and staff nurses; the records of the student nurses were so diverse and the overlapping of nurse training schemes within some groups of hospitals such that it would have been impossible to measure the stability or wastage of their student nurses. The records of the ward sisters and their qualified helpers were, at first sight, more promising; the date of entry into the hospital of each of these was recorded in the minutes and a sample of these was checked with the hospital finance officers. Nevertheless, it was difficult to estimate the mean length of stay, even of the qualified ward staff alone, by this method; our experience at the first five hospitals, described in chapter 2, had already suggested this. To collect the statistics of staff turnover where the range of individual stay may be from two months to 20 years or more demands sampling over a considerable period and our research team had not the resources in manpower to do this thoroughly.

Our second decision was to fall back on establishment ratios, that is, the extent to which the hospital strength is maintained; if, in a given hospital, the complement of sisters, junior sisters and staff nurses on the wards, theatres and other units was, suppose, 40 in all, and if, in January, the number actually in the hospital was 32, this ratio would be 80 per cent. The figure varied from time to time, even from month to month, but the average for the year could be readily computed. We therefore accepted as a measure of staff stability the establishment percentage; this is, admittedly, not a linear function of the mean length of stay of the sisters, but it must be positively correlated with it, if we consider enough sisters and enough hospitals. It is true that the time taken by advertisement and interview in filling a vacant post probably varies between hospitals and is bound to influence the establishment ratio: this must in turn reduce the correlation of staff stability with it. But a list of names of any 15 hospitals written down in rank order of wastage of sisters (and of other qualified ward staff) must look very like that of the same hospitals written down in order of their establishment ratios, but turned upside down. Certainly, most prospective matrons would find it hard to choose between the offer of a post at one hospital with the ward sisters generally at two-thirds of establishment, and at another where few sisters would stay more than two years. If, though we heard it only as expressions of opinion, sisters move towards certain hospitals because their friends are there or advise them to go there; and if, as is certain, sisters move out of other hospitals because they find themselves unable to settle there, it would appear that the hospital that the sisters do not like would be short of staff for both reasons: it would have plenty of resignations and few recommendations. The argument is no stronger than this; we have made no statistical study of the relationship, from one hospital to the next, between mean stay or qualified ward staff and the corresponding establishment ratio. Nevertheless, we have been able to rank the 15 hospitals by this single parameter, called here Q.

Perception, staff stability, and patient stay

The other parameters measured are two of those described in chapter 7; the first is the sisters' perception, averaged over the hospital, of the approachability of their superiors, P; the second is the sisters' attitude towards the integration of their student nurses, K. It is these together that may be taken to suggest the 'atmosphere of the ward'. The array of 15 hospitals by the five measured parameters is set out in Table 8.1. Before discussing the significance of this, it may be desirable to emphasize that the research team, since they collected the statistics, are aware of their shortcomings. The attitude parameters, P and K, are, for example, determined for only a sample of all the sisters in the hospitals; these samples are, however, never less than two-thirds of the total number of sisters on the hospital roll. The estimates of P and K, were made but once; they were not averaged over a year as were Q, M and S, so that some sisters who had left by the end of the year in which Q, M and S were estimated may not have contributed to P and K. These are a few of the objections that can be levelled at any attempt to find statistical relationships among these five measures. Yet it is highly unlikely that these randomizing influences would conspire to make any effect that we are seeking easier to find; experiments relying upon any correlation between identifiable factors are made less, not more, sensitive by contaminating influences, unless the contamination itself is also strongly loaded into both or all of the identifiable factors.

We have ranked the 15 hospitals in this table from A to O according to the sum of the ranks of the five parameters; this varies from 10 to 68. The random probability that, over the array as a whole, the small numbers in the five columns

Table 8.1

Rank orders of 15 acute general hospitals for the parameters set out below.

Hospital	Rank order by five parameters				
	P	K	Q	M	S
A	1	5	2	1	1
B	2	1	9	2	3
C	7	6	1	5	6
D	4	3	12	8	2
E	3	2	6	6	14
F	6	4	7	7	7
G	8	12	3	4	9
H	5	10	5	14	13
I	14	11	10	3	10
J	13	15	4	12	4
K	11	9	13	9	8
L	9	13	8	11	11
M	12	7	15	13	5
N	15	8	11	10	12
O	10	14	14	15	15

P   Sisters' opinions of senior staff
K   Sisters' attitudes towards student nurses
Q   Stability of qualified nursing staff on wards
M   Mean length of patient stay; general medical
S   Mean length of patient stay; general surgical

Coefficient of concordance, $W = 0.51$; significant at 0.1 per cent.

will be associated as they are, and vice versa, is about one in a thousand; in statistical jargon, the coefficient of concordance is 0.51 and this is significant at approximately 0.1 per cent. We must, therefore, conclude that the five parameters are to an appreciable extent related, in spite of the fact that certain hospitals, as, for example, J, show a perverse choice of both low and high rankings. The table confirms, as we should expect, a significant positive correlation between P and K, the two attitudes of the sisters; and a positive correlation between M and S, although it is significant only at 8 per cent. Nevertheless we know from other and more detailed examples, that M and S are, when considered each as made up of many separate diagnostic groups, significantly correlated. The weak element in the concordance of Table 8.1 is Q, although even so this is positively correlated with the other four parameters, and the significance levels with P and M are 10 per cent and 8 per cent respectively. This confirms our interview material with the ward sisters, who frequently remarked that high turnover rate among the patients, on the one hand, and the approval of their consultants, on the other, were the two rewards worth having, and so would make the hospital that had them to offer a place to be worked in. Put in this way, the proposition is not in need of support from statistical evidence, itself none too strong. Yet the free interviews with the sisters, in which they volunteered such remarks, were held in a few hospitals only, and it is of value to find more general support for these associations in a wider sample of hospitals.

The estimates, within the 15 hospitals of this sample, made of the sisters' attitudes to their superiors, P, and to their subordinates, K, are not only significantly correlated with each other at 1 per cent (as we have shown in other hospitals), but they are also correlated with the mean length of patient stay of the medical patients. The correlation of sisters' attitudes towards the integration of the student nurses, K, and the mean period of stay of medical patients, M, is significant at 5 per cent. If we assume that medical patients are, on the whole, more dependent upon the communication system of the ward than are the surgical, it would follow that sisters' attitudes to students would be reflected in the mean stay of the medical patients more than in the mean stay of the surgical, since the sisters' attitudes to their subordinates would determine the amount of information passed, not only to the physicians, but also to the paramedical units upon which the diagnosis and treatment of the medical patient so much depends. It would also affect the solicitude that the student nurse would show to the patients and this may be an ingredient in recovery more vital to the medical patients than to the surgical. We return to this point below, but Table 8.1 suggests that the length of stay of medical patients is more strongly loaded with the hospital factor than any of the four other parameters.

We can use these not entirely surprising conclusions to speculate upon the qualities of 'good' hospitals. There is some evidence to suggest that hospitals able to retain their staffs are also able to discharge their patients more rapidly. While we do not know how to measure the absolute standard of patient care (largely because we have not yet dedicated enough resources to asking what it may be) and so are unable to judge either the condition in which a patient is discharged from hospital or the amount of benefit that he has derived from having been in there, we may ask whether, over large numbers of patients, in comparable areas and identical diagnostic groups, hospitals with short durations of stay differ in any observable particular from hospitals with long; the particulars of greatest interest would be any that suggest the level of patient care provided in the hospital.

Need to determine nature of patient care

It would be of value, for a deeper understanding of many hospital problems, to study certain inter-hospital differences apart from those here discussed. We should know more than we do about, for example, the extent to which the medical staff consult each other over unusual or difficult cases, and how, if at all, they keep in touch with the general practitioners who have sent them; we should know the differing degrees to which the staffs of different hospitals use the services of their ancillary departments, order post-mortem examinations and employ such indirect facilities as the medical library. There is also a vast field for the objective study of nurse–patient interactions at the bedside; 50 normal manual workers between 25 and 35 years of age will remain eight days on average, in hospital X when undergoing appendicectomy; 50 normal manual workers between the same age limits will, for the same operation, remain 12 days in hospital Y, less than 20 miles away. In what observable respects do their experiences in hospital differ? What occupies the 100 hours by which one average duration exceeds the other? We do not know the answers to these conundrums. It has often been remarked to the writer that it is obvious, or that it stands to reason, that the extra four days that, on average, these patients spend in hospital Y must bring to them benefits denied to their counterparts discharged so unfeelingly soon from hospital X. These are obscure subjects on which to advance definite opinions, and it would be well to have evidence to support them. For the present it is hardly possible to go beyond such an argument as this:

'Suppose that hospital X, by forcing the pace of treatment, put the appendicectomies under some disadvantage from which those at hospital Y may be considered free. Then, since it has been shown that the duration of stay not only of appendicectomies, but of all other patients in hospital X will tend to be shorter than that of their counterparts in hospital Y, it would appear that patients in all diagnostic groups at X would suffer something of the same (supposed) disadvantage. If we examine, in otherwise comparable hospitals, those diagnostic groups in which, it may be presumed, the patients respond most variedly to their hospital treatment according to the three different channels of disposal open to them (namely, death, discharge home or transfer to another hospital), we should expect that the hospitals with a significantly short stay for patients discharged home also secure responses in the other classes of disposal less favourable than the hospitals that keep those discharged home significantly longer.'

But what, for example, is meant by suggesting that hospitals might be comparable? Even although particular diagnostic groups are compared only among themselves between comparable hospitals, what evidence is there that the average condition of the patients who enter one hospital is not different from that of those who enter another? The quality of the district nursing services may differ, or the general practitioners in one particular town, for example, may encourage patients with malignant neoplasms to enter the local hospital at a significantly earlier state of the disease than those in another; this would make both the survival rate higher and justify a shorter mean duration of stay among the patients entering that hospital with that complaint, since their average need for treatment would seem to be less. (The hospital that had these satisfactory relationships with local general practitioners would, in the sense of this essay, have a good communication system. The consultants who encouraged this precautionary behaviour among their external colleagues would also be likely to have good relationships with their subordinates inside the hospital.) But it follows that, since there is a significant concordance between average duration of stay by hospitals in all diagnostic groups, this argument (or one producing the same effect) would have to apply not only to malignant neoplasms, but to heart diseases, to pneumonia, to diseases both of the central nervous system and of the digestive system; these five diagnostic groups were found to account for over 70 per cent of the deaths in a sample of 11 hospitals whose records were kindly

69

supplied by the statisticians of a Regional Hospital Board. They are presented in Appendix 8 (page 108) and show, as we would expect, a highly significant concordance between the average durations of stay for these five diagnostic groups.

Other channels of disposal in contrasting hospital groups

The 11 hospitals, which are of different sizes, may then be divided into two classes: Class S, of the four hospitals with the shorter average stays, totalling 1670 beds, and Class L, the seven remaining, totalling 1586 beds. The classification has been made in this way to divide the total bed capacity roughly into two equal sub-totals. The ratio of patients per bed (in these five serious groups) averaged over the year is greater in Class S, by 4·33 to 3·09. Nevertheless, the transfer rate to other hospitals is significantly less in Class S, and when one asks whether there is any detectable difference between the survival rates of the patients who enter Class S hospitals, on the one hand, and those who enter Class L, on the other, the answer is that no clear pattern emerges. If the average total amount of effective care received by a patient discharged home in a hospital of Class S is less than that received by a similar patient in a hospital of Class L, because he has not stayed in there for so long, the factors that make for this deprivation have not, it seems, affected the mean chances of survival, since this is greater in Class S than in Class L. It may not be difficult to suggest reasons for this negative result, apart from those already mentioned, such as that, in spite of observable similarities, the hospitals are not in fact comparable, or that the average admissions at different hospitals are at significantly different stages of affliction with the diseases. For example, to send hopeless cases home to die after only a few days in hospital would both inflate the (apparent) survival rate and reduce the average duration of stay; to persevere with them at the hospital and see them eventually die would reduce the (apparent) survival rate without necessarily affecting the duration of stay of those discharged home, unless patients with a high chance of recovery were sent home rapidly to make beds available for the hopeless cases whose durations of stay were being prolonged. Two consultants in the same hospital who followed these different strategies might therefore both contribute to shortening the average duration of stay, although the efforts of the first cancelled those of the second in their incidence upon the survival rate. Many other speculations are available.

We are not on firm ground in suggesting that the appendicectomies of hospital X, by being there only eight days, have been deprived of something that was vouchsafed in 12 days to their counterparts in hospital Y, and in the absence of firm evidence it is wise to do two things. We should, first, encourage the detailed ward study that alone will enable us to define what we mean by patient care, and, if possible, to assess the extent to which different hospitals provide it. We should, secondly, proceed in the belief that, until evidence can be produced to the contrary, the hospitals that, in the sense of this present chapter, have the shorter average durations of stay are, when comparing like with like, doing no less for their patients than those having the longer. They are, in fact doing a great deal more for those who have not yet been admitted to their wards, by significantly reducing their waiting lists.

The hospital as a learning mechanism

We must ask, therefore, why it is that some hospitals take 12 days to do what others can do in eight days. Since we have no evidence to suggest that the staffs of some hospitals are any more professionally competent than those of others, always excepting the occasional genius whose impression upon a particular hospital outlives him by a generation, there must be some quality of organization that certain hospitals possess to a degree significantly different from that of others. Table 8.1 of this chapter suggests that sisters' attitudes, ward-staff stability and duration of stay are, in some way or other, associated with this quality. This is, in our view, the extent to which the system known as the hospital is able to give to the persons who work in it the information, including the interpretations thereof, that they need to do their work. To the extent that a hospital brings rapid, accurate and useful information to those whose effort requires it, so will that hospital be a good one; where the staff of a hospital know what they are supposed to do or are able to find out what to do; or, in the absence of exact information, can with confidence assess the risks that they are obliged to take, this hospital will tend to display two favourable responses. First, the staff will wish to stay there; secondly, the patients will recover more quickly. The organic quality of the hospital is the transparency of its communications.

The adjustment of the student nurse is evidently a learning process, and since she is called a student it is clear to most people that she has a major need to learn. But it is not so evident that the whole hospital is, or should be, a gigantic learning mechanism and that every act of every person in it contains, or should contain, a significant element of learning. If we may repeat an obvious truism, hospitals *are* different from most other institutions because they deal essentially in human life and health, and it is an observable fact that no two patients are alike, even if they are both Lancashire weavers of the same age, build and habits, with hernias clinically indistinguishable: they are not only different persons both in the eyes of Almighty God as well as in the more prosaic coordinates of their domestic lives, but they react differently to the same nurses on the same ward of the same hospital, and these nurses, in turn, react differently towards each of them. Each patient presents a learning problem to each nurse, to each sister; and each nurse presents each patient with a fresh learning problem in her turn. Just as the doctor has to learn what is wrong with the patient, and perhaps rely upon the nurses to help him with his lessons (especially with medical patients), so will the patient have to learn to adjust himself to life on the ward where he is to be treated. The important element in these vital processes of exchanging information, modifying perceptions, integrating previous experiences and so forth is to perceive and to interpret the effects of one's own activities; learning is the process whereby all in the situation, doctor, nurse and patient alike, are able to find the answers to their own questions. Learning, or adjustment, occurs when, by being enabled to follow the train of one's own doubts or questionings, one can recognize or supplement the contradictory and incomplete patterns of one's existing consciousness. Learning does not occur when one is merely to carry out the instructions dictated by a superior, and in a hospital situation it is impossible beyond narrow limits to lay down universal instructions that suit all patients and all conditions, let alone all consultants and all sisters. Learning, which is the key to the continuous adjustment essential for student nurse and patient alike, may be defined as helping to solve one problem in a way that enables the learner to deal better with the next problem by himself. Every nurse, every sister, every doctor will talk about 'good patients' and 'bad patients'. But they do not all mean the same thing; to some sisters it is the 'good' patient who spends his time in the ward in a state of terrified submission, not daring to ask about his condition, much less to question the logic of his routines. (It would not surprise members of the research team to learn that in some hospitals the patients are able to face the prospect of death with greater composure than can the patients in others.) Such patients must learn little, though they may be subjected to much. To other sisters the 'good' patient is one who asks intelligent questions and who, by trying to understand both his condition and his treatment, is able to accelerate the process of his own recovery, not least by being reassured on some of the grosser fears conjured up by his fevered imagination. We have not yet, alas, been able to study the attitudes of patients, but we have little doubt, in the 12-day hospital we have been discussing, the ward sisters would have a view of a 'good' patient significantly different from that of the sisters in the eight-day hospital of an adjacent town, and we believe that the patients would reflect and amplify these differences. In terms of the hospital as an organism, the 'good' patients of the eight-day hospital would be those who wanted, to the best of their ability, to learn how to participate in their recovery and hence who both generated and absorbed information that enabled the nurses and the doctors also to learn; the 'good' patients in a 12-day hospital, on the other hand, would be those who conformed to the ethic of unquestioning obedience, and who, in not perplexing the nurses or doctors with questions in their own clumsy and unprofessional language, withheld thereby the information enabling the staff to understand the patients better, to diagnose their conditions more keenly and even to recruit them as intelligent members of the teams pledged to their own recovery.

The social dependence of medical patients

There is no evidence to support these speculations, and they must remain the subjective results of our studies. But there is a significant statistical result, set out in Appendix 7 (page 104), that lends additional colour to this concept of a hospital characteristic helping to determine the recovery of the patients. Consider again the broad distinction between medicine and surgery; subject to qualifications, it may be said that the physician must rely more upon reading signs than must the surgeon; he must at times have at his disposal so fleeting and yet so complex a pattern of information as to be taking decisions almost upon his intuition. There is, for example, little in the diagnostic processes of the physician that compares with so decisive an act as opening a patient to the inspection of the surgeon; when he is trying to treat the same condition as the surgeon, such as a peptic ulcer, there must always remain some uncertainty in the mind of the physician about the progress of the case. There are, on this account, patients in certain diagnostic groups who depend upon communications between physician, nurse and other departments of the hospital to a degree altogether more marked than patients in certain other diagnostic groups. Nor.is this all, the progress of the patients in those groups that demand good communications also depends more upon the quality of the nursing; we have shown that the sisters' attitudes to her subordinates reflect the impressions made upon her by her superiors. The solicitude with which the nurses treat their patients is therefore closely bound up with the attitude and communication pattern of the ward; since the pattern on any ward is influenced by a hospital factor, we should expect to find the diagnostic groups treated by the physicians more sensitive to this factor than those treated by the surgeons. In simple language, the average physician is more socially dependent, both for his diagnoses and for the success of his treatment, than is the average surgeon. (This is not contradicted by the demonstration in chapter 3 that length of patient stay of surgical cases in a given diagnostic group in a particular hospital is independent of the consultant.) We must therefore expect that, in the same hospitals, the lengths of stay of patients in each medical group are more strongly influenced by the hospital factor than are the lengths of stay of patients in each surgical group. In the sample of 12 general hospitals that we have been able to examine, in which information has been given of the length of stay of all patients discharged home, we find that the correlation between medical group averages is significantly greater than that between surgical. In other words, it is possible to demonstrate that patients in the six following diagnostic groups:

(a) allergic, endocrine, metabolic and nutritional diseases,
(b) diseases of the central nervous system,
(c) diseases of the heart,
(d) pneumonia,
(e) other diseases of the respiratory system and
(f) other diseases of the digestive system,

are more affected by hospital characteristics, for good or for ill, to shorten or to lengthen their stays, than are patients in another six main diagnostic groups treated in the same hospital; these others are, by and large, less dependent upon the social skills of doctors and nurses alike. The other diagnostic groups are:

(g) appendicitis,
(h) hernia of the abdominal cavity,
(i) diseases of the bones and organs of movement,
(j) benign neoplasms,
(k) diseases of male genitals,
(l) diseases of female genitals.

This statistical result, set out in Appendix 7 (page 105), gives support to the claims so often made by the sisters on medical wards that they are the 'real' nurses, and that it is their skills, both in observing the patient and tending for his needs, no less than those of the doctors, that make for his recovery. Since the deployment of these skills is strongly influenced by the tone of the organic unity with which the hospital is endowed by its communication system, it follows that, in hospitals where this system is opaque, the progress of all medical patients will tend to be retarded, whatever their diagnostic group; where the communication system is lucid all medical patients will tend, whatever their disease, to progress rapidly. The surgical and other patients, on the contrary, while responsive also to the general tone of the hospital, will not show so great a unanimity, since their fates are more in the hands of the individual specialists by whom they are treated. It is remarkable that this significant result can be found in statistics not specifically prepared for this research, and an eloquent illustration of the tenacity and pervasiveness of these social influences.

9. The autotherapeutic organism

We have tried to show that the interactions between the nurse, the patient and the hospital in which they find themselves are simultaneously both complex and simple. We repeat the general argument here in order to introduce suggestions for improving our understanding of these interactions, and so, perhaps, eventually eliminating some of the less desirable results that they produce.

The hospital is an organism characterized by anxiety. Anxiety is enhanced by uncertainty. Uncertainty is magnified by communication failure. Unrealistic ideas about one's own role, knowledge, intelligence, status and other features of the self will increase the difficulties of communicating and of being communicated with. Anxiety, in turn, may inhibit communication through fear of threatening consequences. A regenerative process may start: anxiety, uncertainty, communication blockage, *anxiety, uncertainty, communication blockage,* ANXIETY, UNCERTAINTY, COMMUNICATION BLOCKAGE, etc. But if anxiety is present throughout the hospital, so also is the need to learn. Those who do not know, yet must control the world around them, need to learn. But learning depends upon the very exchange of the information that communication failure suppresses; the greater the anxiety the less is the possibility of the learning that alone can remove the anxiety.

The hospital is an organism endowed with many social systems; the official flow of information and reports is but one of these. For the purpose of this essay this system may be regarded as that which keeps the senior staff of the hospital in touch with, and hence, it is to be hoped, ready to treat the events and emergencies of the wards. It is designed by those in authority to inform and instruct those in authority, so that they may perceive from hour to hour what they should do; this official reporting system is for them a learning mechanism, to remove doubts, to increase knowledge, to test impressions, to resolve arguments, to verify theories, to permit choice, to guide decision, to fortify personal security, to consolidate status, to provide legal evidence and, above all, to respond in whatever way those in charge of it may demand. If this system needs improvement, should it fail to satisfy those who use it as their principal medium of information and learning, it will be amended. In practice, continuous thought will be given by those in authority to these affairs; the system of reporting or of control will be tightened whenever faults are discovered and new checks will be introduced when old methods are found to be wanting. And all this has one main purpose alone: that those in charge may be kept informed and free of doubt, or simply to learn.

There is no corresponding aid for those whose needs to learn are yet greater: the nurse and her patient. Their needs do not require to be repeated in detail; it is enough to say that their entire processes of adjustment to hospital life, whether to stay in the profession or to get better in the bed, are substantially processes of learning, and to repeat that nurses and patients alike do not learn when they are merely told what others think is good for them. Mankind is not just taught; it learns. It learns when, at its own desire and in its own way, it reorganizes its own knowledge. The hospital system is not officially designed to make this readily possible for those in subordinate positions, and the extent to which it happens to be possible is the extent to which the hospital is, in this sense, unofficial, informal, unconventional. The task in hand is to encourage certain hospitals to become, in this sense, less official, less authoritarian, less code-ridden.

This problem is also essentially a learning problem. Those within the hospital, or at least a majority of them, must perceive that their subordinates, in order to learn, must be permitted to make unprogrammed demands upon their superiors. These demands, moreover, may be expected to disturb or even threaten; they may come at times inconvenient to the senior; they may question, even if unintentionally, the authority, knowledge, judgement or values of the senior; they may bring to the senior facts or interpretations of facts that he or she would prefer not to recognize; they may suggest a need for change in the senior, change that might be not merely difficult but painful.

It is quite evident that, if such learning is desirable, it will not come about by exhortation. It is of no use merely to point out to any particular hospital that it has an abnormally high nurse wastage rate and a mean length of patient stay significantly longer than the average for others of a comparable class, and that these, in the perception of outsiders, will be reduced only when communications are improved. For the very communication difficulties that have brought with them these disabling effects will prevent the organism from assessing its own vision; general arguments about nurse wastage will be countered by remarks about the poor quality of local recruits; general arguments about length of patient stay exceeding the average will be met by remarks about the high quality of treatment given in return. These responses we know from experience.

In some hospitals it may be possible to effect improvement by purely institutional methods. Specific administrative steps may help, such as setting up consultative committees between different levels or classes of staff, but they will make progress only if there is a collective will to do so; if they are not supported in this way from the start, they may do positive harm and give existing isolationisms or animosities a new dimension. It might, conceivably, make student nurses or cadets more at home in the hospital to attach each of them to a personal tutor, who might or might not be a member of the teaching staff; there is no reason why a ward or departmental sister should not be the established confidant of half a dozen junior nurses if the staff of the training school is overburdened with official duties. This system of nominating a senior member of the staff as the personal adviser or tutor of each junior nurse could, although with

76

difficulty, it is true, be extended to those classes of patient whose stay in the hospital was likely to exceed, say, two whole weeks. It has recently been suggested that the medical staff should undertake these very duties. These and other ways of establishing channels of information designed to help all subordinates to learn will occur to any student of hospital organization whose attention is drawn to the need.

It is, however, questionable whether by themselves they would produce much improvement. True communication lies not so much in the physical passage of information, as, for example, through telephone systems and on hospital forms carried by messengers, as it lies in the will to communicate and in the desire to know whether the communication is serving the needs of those who seek it. A personal tutor must make a positive effort, personal to herself, not only to find out what is the problem of her student—and the student may not, at the outset, know her problem any more clearly than the patient knows his illness; a tutor must also go to great pains to understand her personal relations to the student and her own motivations behind any advice that she may care to offer her. This self knowledge, if, but only if, it is sought by being desired, can be gained by appropriate exercises in group dynamics; there is no doubt that methods of social psychotherapy, such as are being developed in America by the National Training Laboratories and in Britain by the Tavistock Institute, have considerable promise in the hospital service generally. Their success, however, will probably be bound up with the future success, if any, of social psychology in the wider field of medical education.

There is, however, an urgent need for therapeutic methods of a more direct, if less sophisticated, nature, merely to advance the cultural preparation by which these exercises in group dynamics must, if they are to succeed, be heralded. It is essential to engender within many of the hospital staffs as they now exist this concept of an organic unity, of a mutual dependence and of the necessity for each individual to perceive more clearly his or her role in the total process. Where this concept of the organism is lacking, and the hospital suffers from parataxis, a major learning effort is called for, but this should be attempted only if there is a common desire to succeed in it. Those in the confused situation should set out to improve their relationships only if they want to do so. This desire is partly an emotional, partly an intellectual drive, and it is impossible to suggest in general terms, that is, without detailed local study, whether it might already exist, or could be engendered, in any particular hospital. Even if, in some way, a collective will to improvement could be identified there might still be substantial problems in canalizing it.

Yet our researches suggest that there are, or may be, reasonably straightforward ways of tackling these problems. Our excursions into the methods of general attitude surveys show that interesting patterns of problems can be traced in different hospitals. The data of Table 6.1 (a), (b) and (c) can be rearranged by subject of comment to show that such-and-such a problem may be of great concern to large numbers of persons within the hospital. The problem may involve different departments, from operating theatre to medical records, and different levels of authority, from consultants to porters; whatever it may be, the attitude survey brings it into the open, identifying, too, any anxiety that it may create, with all the emphasis of detail revealed by the aerial photograph of an overgrown Roman encampment. Problems that are brought out in this way are, of course, usually felt by the hospital administration; it would be presumptuous to suggest, for example, that the hospital secretary might be unaware of stresses within the patient-movement system, or that the matron was not already uneasy about her need to fill the nursing establishment with many auxiliaries simply because there was a lack of students. This is not the point. However painful the problem may be, the hospital is in no position to deal with it unless it has a clear view of the effects it has upon those who suffer under it. For a hospital secretary to say that he is aware of a patient-movement problem is one thing; to take therapeutic action is another. To know that one is unwell is an experience granted to us all at some time or another; to know our precise trouble and what to do to put it right are quite different things. To know that one's village is the site of a Roman settlement is one thing; to trace its ramifications and access roads by aerial reconnaissance is quite another. The attitude survey, if properly carried out, amplifies the impressions of those in authority at the hospital to a comparable degree.

It should not be difficult, given the pattern of anxiety aroused by particular problems at a particular hospital, to seek some kind of cure or treatment for one or more of them. If widespread concern about patient-movement has been voluntarily expressed by a large number of those involved in moving patients, it may be assumed that they feel an emotional drive to help improve the system; our studies show that in attitude surveys the first comments volunteered are about matters on which the staff would like action to be taken. The desire to improve the situation is there, and may add up to a substantial social force; the problem is then to bring this force intelligently to bear. This is the precise field of the operational research worker, with his systematic approach to the delineation of complex problems, with his analysis of statistical data, his measurements of work tasks, his mapping of procedures and his reduction of processes and methods to their elements. It would be an advance of the first magnitude to make freely available to the hospital service the services or advice of a few teams of operational research workers.

But the hospital presents special problems and the operational research worker has still an apprenticeship to serve within the hospital. For within industry, where his success is now widely acknowledged, he is normally the adviser or the agent of the most senior level of authority; he draws his powers from the Board, he makes his recommendations to the Board and, if the Board approve them, it is the Board that put them into effect. In practice, the Board may well seek his advice upon their possible impact, but he is the servant of the policy makers and he is there primarily to improve their grasp. In the hospital the main problems, as they are argued in this essay, are not those of policy; the nurses, the sisters, the doctors, the paramedical staff, the porters and domestics are at one with the hospital management committee and with each other; all are agreed that their collective task is to help the patients to the greatest extent within their capacity. There is, unlike in most industrial and commercial concerns, no conflict between their value systems; it is over their different perceptions of the hospital problems that the conflicts arise. The confusion is not strategic but tactical; it is not about the tasks that need to be done, but about the manner of their doing. The operational research worker is thus to be regarded as a servant or colleague of the staff rather than as an agent of the superior administration. His task, moreover, is as much to identify the perception that different members of the staff hold of their roles and of their part in the total problem under review as it is to delineate any objective problem itself. It thus follows that a team set on to assist this process of social learning will need to command a significant understanding of the psychology of perception. Nor is this all. As far as possible the collection, interpretation and use of whatever data may seem to be needed for the solution or amelioration of the problem in hand should be carried out by the staff largely affected by that problem. The perception and attitudes of ordinary persons are not altered merely because somebody produces intellectual arguments, however sound, in favour of such alteration; these processes of change, if they are to succeed at all, demand constant interaction between the subject and the surroundings that he is encouraged to reassess. The essence of this interaction, which is the foundation of all learning, is the feedback loop by which the subject becomes aware of his own effect upon the situation, and of the effect that the situation has upon him. It is by this feedback loop that the child learns his mother tongue, by observing, interpreting and employing the responses that are made by those around him to his baby utterances; these early lessons he will remember more tenaciously than the expensive and laborious efforts of later life, when other parties, in the form of teachers, try to impose upon him a foreign language. Indeed, to attempt any fundamental change, or learning, mainly through the medium of a third party or, even more so, to press down upon the subject by the weight of authority alone some new programme of rules intended to modify the behaviour, in the hope that values, perceptions, attitudes and similar determinants of personal conduct are susceptible to purely external manipulation, are alike unprofitable exercises. Only by working through problems that have for the subject a strong emotional content is there any possibility of modifying his or her role-perception and hence of diminishing the amount of parataxis from which the hospital may suffer. 'Working through the problem' is, of course, a complex process; some members of staff may be involved more deeply than are others; some may be well placed to collect or interpret such-and-such facts, others may find it more rewarding to attempt this part of the solution rather than that. In trying to organize the collective desire of those at the hospital to see some part of its system improved, the operational research team will need to secure many agreements from those in authority about the depth and nature of the participation that they might subscribe from the various members of staff. We have a great deal to learn in preparation for this activity; we must, in particular, be realistic enough to recognize that these experiments in social therapy are going to appear as a threat to some senior officers. 'If', some hospital secretary will say, 'you discover by your attitude surveys—the results of which, in any case, I do not accept, because how can you possibly know whether people are telling you the truth?*—that patient movement creates as much widespread anxiety as you suggest—and you are not telling me anything I don't know already—surely the *right* thing to do is to let the management committee decide what ought to be done about it? After all, they are in charge of the hospital, aren't they? Surely you agree that those in charge must put it right? . . .' It would be impossible to attempt this form of social education in such a hospital until the attitude of the secretary had itself been modified.

Yet, in the opinion of at least one observer, the biggest difficulty is not in the upper ranks of the hospital administration; there are, on the contrary, many people in the Ministry, at the offices of the Regional Boards and among the Hospital Management Committees who would be willing to see radical experiments undertaken in the field of attitudinal change, and to give them their personal approval and even financial support. One of the less visible benefits of the nationalization of the hospitals has been, in a few imaginations at least, a more structured view of their human problems. The obstacles to success in the kind of programme suggested here are rather our lack of experience in how to apply these methods of social therapy in institutions as fraught with anxiety as are hospitals; and, perhaps more so, the extreme shortage of operational research workers knowledgeable in these affairs. The protests of those to whom all learning, all change, all progress is but a scandalous corruption of some golden past may still attract applause, but there are at many strategic points in the hospital service those who recognize the need for and will support new approaches. It remains to be seen whether their patience will be rewarded throughout the long and difficult research processes necessary to finding those who can undertake these studies, and who themselves must slowly learn the methods best suited to effect the changes.

One thing is clear. The hospitals themselves, personified by their administrators, their doctors and their nurses, must actively join these studies, and members of these professions must learn to conduct surveys, to interpret their findings, to seek the structure of the problems so revealed and to build the programmes of participation by which these problems may be ameliorated. There is no lack of goodwill or of first-class human material; at all levels in the service there are those for whom a cooperative study of this type would be one of the most rewarding contributions to their career development. It is at present a question of how such researches can best be done and how the universities and the hospital professions can cooperate. A hesitating start is being made; it will eventually succeed. But change can be no faster than the hospital service can envision, and no faster than the research workers can themselves stumble forward. We are now only getting ready at the starting post; what race is to be run we do not yet perceive. This we can be sure of: the going will be hard, yet, although some of the spectators will be hostile, the prizes will be well worth winning.

* This usually means: 'In situations of complete freedom of expression, where there are no fears for the consequences, I personally should not know whether to tell the truth or not.'

Appendix 1
Nurse sickness rates as hospital characteristics

Table 1.2 reveals significant differences between hospitals in overall sickness-absence rates among student nurses. These may be due to differences in levels of medical attention or merely to differences between the reporting or recording systems. It is interesting to see the reported sickness rates increase from A to C and then decrease from C to E. This trend, first up and then down, appears to be significant, or associated with the various hospitals. Is the pressure of disapproval in hospitals D and E such that it is regarded as a weakness for a student nurse to report sick? Table 1.2 may be rewritten in terms of rank orders of sickness-absence rates as Table A1.1 below.

Table A1.1

Class of student nurse	A	B	C	D	E
(a)	1	3	4	5	2
(b)	2	1	5	4	3
(c)	1	2	5	4	3
Sum of ranks	4	6	14	13	8

(Coefficient of concordance = 0·84; significant at 1 per cent.)

In our studies at hospital E we found considerable direct evidence of nurses working under stress; some ought undoubtedly to have been receiving medical attention. Their comment was that it was unendurably depressing to be ill, since the sick room was so miserable a place; and that the nurse obliged to enter it was shown no sympathy and was even denied visitors. It may well be that many student nurses in this hospital eventually responded to a total pattern of treatment, embracing inadequate medical care, by giving up their training altogether. The shoemaker's children grow accustomed to being the worst shod, but there is much to suggest that care of the nurses' health not seldom deserves more attention than it appears to attract.

Appendix 2
Size-effects in hospitals

The hospital service provides some interesting illustrations of size-effects: one of the most curious was noted by Sir James Young Simpson in 1869.

Table A2.1

The risk of death following the amputation of any of the four limbs, by hospitals according to size, 1869.

Size of hospital by no. of beds	No. of limb amputations	No. of deaths	Deaths per 100 amputations
Private houses	2098	226	10·8
Less than 25	143	20	14·0
26–100	761	134	17·6
101–200	1370	310	22·6
201–300	803	228	28·4
Above 300	2089	855	41·0

Source: *B.M.J.*, 1869.

These figures were collected when ideas upon cross-infection were perhaps less in the medical mind than they are said to be today. But it would be rash to assert that this table and Table 1.3 have nothing in common.

Hospital accident rates

A second size-effect is the trend of accident rates as hospitals become larger.

If, as Freud suggests, accidents fulfil the useful purpose of enabling a person to retire from a situation that he does not like, the very marked rise in the employee-injury rate accompanying the increase in size of American hospitals would seem to indicate poor adjustment to the large community. Note that Table A2.2 suggests a higher risk to the individual, not merely a greater total number of accidents simply because there are more employees to suffer them.

Hospital absences

The absence, both for sickness and for other reasons, of hospital staffs as a function of hospital size is interesting. No pattern emerges as long as all hospitals are

Table A2.2

Number of accidents per million employee hours in American hospitals, 1953, by type and size of hospitals.

Size of hospital by no. of employees	Accident rate by type and size of hospital				
	General	Mental	T.B.	Special	All
Below 10	2·5	⎫	⎫ 7·5	2·9	2·6
10–19	2·5	⎬ 6·3	⎬		3·2
20–49	4·1	⎭	9·1	9·3	5·0
50–99	4·5	8·1	7·4	6·7	5·1
100–249	5·3	7·6	8·0	8·6	6·0
250–499	6·2	8·7	12·6	9·5	7·3
500–999	7·4	15·4	16·4	13·4	10·0
1000–2499	8·4	⎫ 21·0	13·8	25·5	13·5
2500 and over	10·3	⎭	—	—	12·4

Source: US Bureau of Labor Statistics.

Table A2.3

Distribution of all staff absences by size of hospital, for all 60 Class 1 hospitals in the same region, 1960.

Size range by no. of full-time staff	No. of hospitals	Full-time staff			Part-time staff		
		Total staff	Total abs.	Av. abs. per person	Total staff	Total abs.	Av. abs. per person
Above 50	16	3282	1030	0·314	652	222	0·340
25–50	22	978	221	0·226	460	164	0·356
Below 25	22	276	54	0·196	150	48	0·320

Table A2.4

Distribution of all staff absences by size of hospital, for all 25 Class 2 hospitals in the same region, 1960.

Size range by no. of staff* employed	No. of hospitals	Full-time staff			Part-time staff		
		Total staff	Total abs.	Av. abs. per person	Total staff	Total abs.	Av. abs. per person
Above 50	4	189	66	0·349	338	209	0·618
25–30	7	143	22	0·154	221	56	0·253
Below 25	14	102	27	0·265	180	39	0·217

* The number of staff for setting the size class is taken to be the sum of all full-time plus half of the part-time staff.

considered together, but when they are considered as two distinct classes, those in which there are more full-time staff than part-time, and vice versa, an interesting pattern is revealed. One of the Regional Hospital Boards which takes a special interest in its statistical services has supplied the data of Tables A2.3 and A2.4. There are 60 hospitals in the region with a predominance of full-time staff (class 1) and 25 with a predominance of part-time (class 2). The full-time staff in the class 1 hospitals and the part-time staff in the class 2 show highly significant size-effects in the absence patterns; there is no such pattern among the part-time employees in class 1 hospitals nor among the full-time staff in class 2.

The trends of increasing absence with increasing size are thus highly significant for full-time staff in class 1 hospitals; and for part-time staff in class 2 hospitals. The larger hospitals with a majority of part-time staff show very high sickness-absence rates; this could be explained on the assumption made throughout this essay, namely, that any effect tending to increase the difficulty of communications tends also to depress morale.

Appendix 3
Differences between lengths of patient stay

Table 3.1 suggests that the average lengths of stay of appendicectomies in seven acute general hospitals differ among themselves; the shortest is 8·3 days, the longest 11·6. The significance of the differences can be demonstrated by analysing the variance of the length of stay among the 654 patients into variance between hospitals and variance within hospitals. Table A3·1 shows the results of this analysis.

Table A3.1

Source of variation	Sum of squares	Degrees of freedom	Estimate of variance	F
Between hospitals	1 144	6	191	
				7·02
Within hospitals	17 588	647	27·2	
Total	18 732	653	28·7	

So large a value of F could have occurred by random chance about once in a million times; we conclude that the differences between the averages are thus not random and must be assigned to real differences between the hospitals. The multi-sample median test is simpler; the 654 lengths of stay are set out in rank order and the median identified. If there were no significant differences between hospital averages, all hospitals would tend to have half of their sample above and half of it below the median; it is easy to calculate whether any tendency for samples not to be equally divided is significant. In the present sample, χ^2, for six degrees of freedom, is about 81, suggesting very significant differences indeed, Similar methods can be employed to test the significance of differences between surgeons or wards in helping to determine the length of stay within any given hospital; no such differences could be found in the sample of seven hospitals and 3000 cases examined.

Appendix 4
Length of patient stay as a hospital characteristic

The following table is formed by putting the entries of Table 3.4 into rank orders, instead of actual days, of duration of stay.

Table A4.1

Rank orders of length of patient stay for 14 hospitals in same region, and for nine diagnostic groups; all patients discharged home.

Hospital	Rank order of length of patient stay by diagnostic groups								
	(a)	(b)	(c)	(d)	(e)	(f)	(g)	(h)	(i)
I	11	3	6	11	11	4	1	1	2
II	$13\frac{1}{2}$	13	9	3	1	1	2	12	14
III	$13\frac{1}{2}$	12	$12\frac{1}{2}$	14	12	13	3	10	9
IV	8	11	7	13	14	$10\frac{1}{2}$	4	3	5
V	7	7	$10\frac{1}{2}$	8	6	$6\frac{1}{2}$	13	7	8
VI	$9\frac{1}{2}$	2	1	7	$8\frac{1}{2}$	3	$8\frac{1}{2}$	2	1
VII	5	4	$3\frac{1}{2}$	2	$2\frac{1}{2}$	5	10	8	6
VIII	6	6	8	1	5	8	6	11	7
IX	4	1	$12\frac{1}{2}$	4	$8\frac{1}{2}$	$10\frac{1}{2}$	5	9	4
X	2	8	2	6	$2\frac{1}{2}$	$6\frac{1}{2}$	12	6	10
XI	$9\frac{1}{2}$	9	5	10	13	9	11	14	12
XII	12	10	$10\frac{1}{2}$	12	10	14	7	13	13
XIII	3	14	14	9	4	12	14	5	11
XIV	1	5	$3\frac{1}{2}$	5	7	2	$8\frac{1}{2}$	4	3

(a) arteriosclerotic heart disease
(b) varicose veins
(c) haemorrhoids
(d) pneumonia
(e) bronchitis

(f) peptic ulcer
(g) appendicitis
(h) hernia repair
(i) diseases of the gall bladder

The sum of the ranks, across the rows, varies from as low as 39 for hospital XIV to as high as $101\frac{1}{2}$ for hospital XII (half marks arise from the sharing of two rank orders in event of a tie). The coefficient of concordance of this array is 0·31. This is significant at one part in a thousand, corresponding to a value of $\chi^2 = 36$ for 13 degrees of freedom; to an unpractised and sceptical eye the table, and Table 3.4 may look quite formless.

The table of rank orders above has, however, been included for another reason. The correlation between rank orders of bronchitis and pneumonia is 0·77, significant at about one part in a thousand, while there is no corresponding correlation between rank orders of appendicectomy and hernia repair. The concordance of the 'surgical' groups as a whole is only just significant, whereas that of the 'medical' is highly so. This point is dealt with more fully in chapter 8 and demonstrated again, in a different sample of hospitals, in Appendix 7.

Appendix 5
The measurement of sisters' attitudes

1. In chapter 7 we suggest that the attitudes of ward sisters towards the integration of their student nurses are dependent upon their perceptions of the attitudes of their own superiors rather than upon the sisters' own commitment on questions of hierarchy and status. We base our argument upon measurement and correlation in the following way.

2. Suppose that the 12 attitudes that we attempt to assess are set forth in the following specific statements (see Appendix 5a):

(a) About integration and training
(i) Sister can devote time to instructing the student nurse only at the expense of what may be more important demands.
(ii) Conferences of the ward staff to discuss their personal or clinical problems are not worth the time they would take up.
(iii) Sisters need not attempt to explain to their subordinates instructions coming down from a higher level.
(iv) A sister who demands a high standard of work from her staff usually makes herself disliked by them.

(b) To hierarchy and status
(v) In planning the ward duty rota, preference for desirable hours and time off should be given according to seniority.
(vi) The tradition that nursing staff of similar status should keep together at mealtimes is essential to the efficiency of the hospital.
(vii) Even on a ward with two or more consultants sister should always deal with them herself.
(viii) Modern developments in clinical practice can succeed only if sister gives more and more time to purely clerical work.

(c) To superiors
(ix) In the doctor/nurse partnership the credit is unfairly divided.
(x) The matron and her administrative staff are no longer as closely in touch with ward problems as they should be.
(xi) Sisters in this hospital are confident that any solutions to their problems reached at their formal meetings will always be put into effect.
(xii) Ancillary departments, such as the pharmacy, kitchen or maintenance,

seem to sister to be organized for their own convenience rather than that of the wards.

3. Sisters were invited, in conditions of secrecy and non-collusiveness, to state to what extent they agreed or disagreed with these remarks. Five alternatives were offered:

(a) strongly agree
(b) agree or tend to agree
(c) uncertain or no opinion
(d) disagree or tend to disagree
(e) strongly disagree.

Where the opinion suggested closeness, ease of contact or positive personal involvement scores of $+2$ or $+1$ were awarded; opinions that suggested aloofness, difficulty of contact or personal disengagement attracted scores of -1 or -2. Thus, agreement with all statements other than (xi) would attract negative marks, disagreements would attract positive marks. The average mark scored by 350 sisters in 15 hospitals was significantly positive in all 12 cases.

Table A5.1

	i	ii	iii	iv	v	vi	vii	viii	ix	x	xi	xii
i		21	27	20	01	03	09	09	23	39	11	15
ii			20	19	03	04	−08	−08	11	37	32	26
iii				15	02	17	−03	−03	08	39	16	18
iv					09	05	05	−07	15	21	12	11
v						19	22	19	07	07	−01	07
vi							15	24	−08	03	00	08
vii								27	06	06	07	13
viii									07	03	−02	06
ix										10	31	29
x											21	30
xi												41
xii												

4. We correlate the scores of all 350 sisters between pairs of statements; from these 12 pairs we find 66 correlation coefficients. They are in fact 66 drawn from a much larger population of 2145 correlation coefficients, since not only the 12 statements above were employed but 54 others as well (see Appendix 5a). These 2145 were normally distributed around a mean of $+0.05$ with standard deviation 0.10. The particular 66 coefficients in which we are interested are set out in Table A5.1 in which decimal points are omitted.

5. If T stands for a collective attitude to the integration of the student nurse, H to hierarchy and P to superiors, Table A5.1 can be expressed as Table A5.2.

Table A5.2

	T	H	P
T H P	0·203 (6)	0·024 (16) 0·210 (6)	0·209 (16) 0·043 (16) 0·270 (6)

In this table the figures in brackets are the numbers of correlation coefficients, whose average value is also given to three figures. It is easy to show that the means of four sets of these coefficients, name TT, TP, HH and PP are significantly greater than the population mean of 0·05 and that the means of HT and HP are not significantly different from that population mean. This conclusion depends only upon the distribution of the correlation coefficients as observed; it does not depend upon the significance of any particular correlation coefficient.

6. The significance of these coefficients cannot be read from ordinary tables as we do not correlate normally distributed bimodal variates. Either can assume one of five discrete values only, namely $+ 2$, $+ 1$, zero, $- 1$ and $- 2$. But a comparison of these coefficients with the tetrachoric correlation coefficient shows that we are safe in testing their significance by the formula $\chi^2 = nr^2$ used with the tetrachoric coefficient. Since $n = 350$ a value of $r = 0·2$ gives $\chi^2 = 14$ for one degree of freedom. This is significant at about 0·02 per cent. It means the chances of the four statements of TT, whose six coefficients average more than 0·20, not displaying some common factor, but reaching this very significant value by pure chance six times (though there are but 3 degrees of freedom), is negligible. These four statements thus belong to a particular family, as one would expect on the grounds of common sense. Likewise with HH and with PP.

7. The cross-correlations of T and P are of the same average order of magnitude. Whatever it is that is common to all T is no less loaded into all P; and vice versa. The mean of the 28 coefficients in the PP, PT and TT blocks is indeed 0·220, which suggests an inner consistency.

8. The 32 correlation coefficients, on the other hand, of the four H-statements and eight of P and T, average, however, only 0·034. This is not significantly different from the population mean and gives us no reason to feel that H is related to either P or T.

9. We conclude from this that the commitment of the ward sisters to hierarchical beliefs is in no way associated with their attitudes to the integration of their junior nurses. On the other hand, there is a significant relationship between their attitudes to the integration of the junior nurses and their perceptions of their own integration into the larger organization of the hospital on which they themselves depend.

10. We can demonstrate this dependence in a more direct fashion. Consider the following statements that reveal once more the attitudes of sisters:

(a) Most young people of today have had too soft an upbringing.

(b) Education today gives the student nurse too much theory.

(c) Sisters can devote time to instructing the student nurse only at the expense of what may be more important demands.

(d) The matron and her administrative staff are no longer as closely in touch with ward problems as they should be.

(e) The medical staff tend to treat suggestions from the nurses with less consideration than they deserve.

(f) Ancillary departments, such as the pharmacy, kitchen and maintenance, seem to sister to be organized for their own convenience rather than that of the wards.

The opinions of 622 ward sisters drawn from 28 hospitals and two conferences were collected on these six statements, and scored as in two blocks, each of three statements. Scores thus ranged from + 6 to − 6 on each block of three statements for any individual sister. The grouping of the statements into two blocks of three was, of course, the first three statements to measure T; the second three to measure P. All sisters can then be classified into four ranges both by their T scores and their P scores as follows.

Attitudes towards T

− 6, − 5, − 4 or − 3	: disparaging
− 2 or − 1	: indifferent
zero or + 1	: aware
+ 2, + 3, + 4, + 5 or + 6	: solicitious

Perceptions of P

− 6, − 5, − 4 or − 3	: hostile
− 2 or − 1	: aloof
zero or + 1	: responsive
+ 2, + 3, + 4, + 5 or + 6	: forthcoming

The distribution of the 622 sisters by these two sets of criteria is given in Table A5.3.

Table A5.3

Distribution of 622 ward sisters by impressions of superiors, P, and by attitudes towards subordinates, T.

T, *or attitudes towards subordinates*	P, *or impression of superiors*			
	Forthcoming	*Responsive*	*Aloof*	*Hostile*
Solicitous	58	42	23	9
Aware	60	47	44	36
Indifferent	32	53	50	41
Disparaging	10	24	36	57

This shows that there is a highly significant association between the impression made upon a ward sister by her superiors and the attitude that she displays towards her subordinates. In simple terms, a ward sister passes on to her nurses the treatment she feels herself to receive from those to whom she is in her turn responsible. The thesis advanced in this essay is that the mechanism of transmission is the degree of tension or anxiety by which the sister is disturbed; this anxiety is a measure, in turn, of the uncertainty that she feels in her task, and this again depends upon the communication system of the hospital; and in particular upon the confidence that she feels in its responses to her needs. If she can, in other words, on her own initiative, get her questions answered or her problems dealt with, she will help her nurses to overcome their own problems, and so to learn.

Appendix 5a
Opinion survey among ward sisters

The following set of printed statements was put simultaneously to the ward sisters of one particular hospital, generally in the relaxed informality of the sisters' lounge. Collusion was always impossible and anonymity was maintained throughout. The percentages entered under each statement give the responses, averaged over about 30 hospitals, of 622 ward sisters. The average time of completion was 20 minutes; two sisters alone refused to fill in the document. The discussions that followed the exercise were always prolonged, vigorous and, for research workers and sisters alike, highly informative.

In this document there are 66 statements.
None are necessarily true; none are necessarily false. They contain no hidden meanings; there are no catches in them. But you will agree or disagree with them to some extent, perhaps strongly, unless you are uncertain what any statement means, or unless you cannot be sure which way the balance lies. Will you please show under each item what your opinion is by putting a ring round the appropriate letters?

SA means strongly agree
 A means agree or tend to agree
 U means uncertain or undecided
 D means disagree or tend to disagree
SD means strongly disagree

Example: Sister should always try to be cheerful.

SA Ⓐ U D SD

1. Sisters cannot do much to improve the morale of their ward staffs since they cannot alter the policies of the hospital.

SA	A	U	D	SD
4%	11%	4%	42%	39%

2. If matron asks a sister to make a change affecting the work of nursing students it is unnecessary for the sister to discuss it with them first.

SA	A	U	D	SD
4%	20%	6%	43%	27%

93

3. Most young people of today have had too soft an upbringing.

SA	A	U	D	SD
10%	30%	19%	37%	4%

4. One of the most important characteristics of a good nurse is the respect she shows for the medical staff.

SA	A	U	D	SD
10%	44%	9%	28%	9%

5. The first principle of good leadership is to issue precise and detailed instructions to one's subordinates.

SA	A	U	D	SD
56%	35%	3%	6%	—

6. Sister is expected to take the view that her immediate superior is always right.

SA	A	U	D	SD
2%	18%	11%	50%	19%

7. It is impossible for a sister to run a ward with a large staff without at times appearing to display favouritism.

SA	A	U	D	SD
—	13%	8%	49%	30%

8. The matron and her administrative staff are no longer as closely in touch with ward problems as they should be.

SA	A	U	D	SD
20%	33%	8%	29%	10%

9. In planning the ward duty rota, preference for desirable hours and time off should be given according to seniority.

SA	A	U	D	SD
9%	37%	6%	39%	9%

10. A sister should use her own judgement about what information to give the patient without consulting the doctor.

SA	A	U	D	SD
5%	33%	8%	38%	16%

11. Ward problems that may concern both matron and the hospital secretary (such as finance or supplies) are generally dealt with quickly and sensibly.

SA	A	U	D	SD
4%	39%	20%	28%	9%

12. Conferences of the ward staff to discuss their personal or clinical problems are not worth the time they would take up.

SA	A	U	D	SD
2%	9%	14%	47%	28%

13. Sisters are given every encouragement to contribute items of business to their regular meetings with matron.

SA	A	U	D	SD
20%	56%	8%	12%	4%

14. The medical staff tend to treat suggestions from the nurses with less consideration than they deserve.

SA	A	U	D	SD
8%	29%	8%	47%	8%

15. Education today gives the student nurse too much theory.

SA	A	U	D	SD
13%	34%	15%	31%	7%

16. There are times when sister should go out of her way to understand the personal problems of her staff.

SA	A	U	D	SD
38%	56%	3%	3%	—

17. A sister who wants to get on in her profession must seek frequent changes of hospital.

SA	A	U	D	SD
10%	28%	19%	38%	5%

18. Parents today do not exercise enough discipline over their children.

SA	A	U	D	SD
23%	47%	19%	10%	1%

19. Sisters in this hospital are confident that any solutions to their problems reached at their formal meetings will always be put into effect.

SA	A	U	D	SD
15%	39%	20%	21%	5%

20. The tradition that nursing staff of similar status should keep together at mealtimes is essential to the efficiency of the hospital.

SA	A	U	D	SD
7%	32%	11%	36%	14%

21. Departments like path. lab., X-ray and medical records always have to be chased to give sister the information she needs.

SA	A	U	D	SD
19%	32%	12%	32%	5%

22. A reprimand is more effective when given in front of others.

SA	A	U	D	SD
—	—	—	31%	69%

23. Ancillary departments, such as the pharmacy, kitchen or maintenance, seem to the sister to be organized for their own convenience rather than that of the wards.

SA	A	U	D	SD
11%	31%	13%	37%	8%

24. Sisters can devote time to instructing the student nurse only at the expense of what may be more important demands.

SA	A	U	D	SD
10%	38%	8%	39%	6%

25. Nurses should not address each other by their Christian names when on duty.

SA	A	U	D	SD
77%	16%	2%	2%	3%

26. Nurses of all ranks feel perfectly free to seek clarification of orders from the consultants themselves.

SA	A	U	D	SD
7%	21%	15%	39%	18%

27. Matron should consult the sisters before changing the work routine of the nursing staff.

SA	A	U	D	SD
54%	43%	1%	2%	—

28. As a matter of principle matrons should always be in charge of hospital housekeeping.

SA	A	U	D	SD
7%	14%	27%	38%	14%

29. It is essential that even the most junior nurse should know all she can about the diagnosis and treatment of her patients.

SA	A	U	D	SD
58%	37%	2%	2%	1%

30. The junior nurse makes little real contribution to the work of the ward before well into her second year.

SA	A	U	D	SD
4%	7%	4%	51%	34%

31. Modern developments in clinical practice can succeed only if sister gives more and more time to purely clerical work.

SA	A	U	D	SD
4%	14%	20%	39%	23%

32. In this hospital sister would make a recommendation about a patient only if the doctor asked her for it.

SA	A	U	D	SD
1%	6%	9%	51%	33%

33. Generally speaking, it is undesirable for junior nurses to accompany the consultant on his ward round.

SA	A	U	D	SD
9%	39%	10%	33%	9%

34. Unquestioned obedience to one's superior is absolutely essential in the hospital.

SA	A	U	D	SD
19%	38%	9%	28%	6%

35. A marked professional distance is kept between the senior medical staff here and those recently qualified.

SA	A	U	D	SD
2%	16%	19%	55%	8%

36. If matron wants to make a change affecting the duties of the nursing staff it is a sign of weakness for her to discuss it with the sisters first.

SA	A	U	D	SD
3%	2%	—	39%	56%

37. Sister should know what the nurse thinks and feels about her work even if she seems to be putting her back into it.

SA	A	U	D	SD
30%	63%	5%	2%	—

38. Only the senior nurse on duty should discuss the patient's condition with a relative.

SA	A	U	D	SD
56%	39%	2%	2%	1%

39. Formal meetings of sisters with the senior staff at this hospital seem little more than somebody laying down the law.

SA	A	U	D	SD
4%	16%	20%	43%	17%

40. Taken over the whole year, sister has very few complaints about getting all the information she needs to run her ward properly.

SA	A	U	D	SD
7%	60%	16%	15%	2%

41. Discipline is impaired if sister has a personal friend among her ward staff.

SA	A	U	D	SD
16%	33%	14%	31%	6%

42. The medical committee always ask the sisters what they think about any changes of practice that will affect nursing care.

SA	A	U	D	SD
8%	43%	17%	26%	6%

43. In the doctor–nurse partnership the credit is unfairly divided.

SA	A	U	D	SD
4%	17%	20%	52%	7%

44. Ancillary departments, like the laundry, kitchen or engineers, do not always realize that they are there primarily to service the wards.

SA	A	U	D	SD
20%	44%	8%	24%	4%

45. Even during her preliminary training the student nurse is still given glamourized ideas of her future work.

SA	A	U	D	SD
4%	18%	10%	58%	10%

46. A good sister will not admit to her staff that she has made a mistake.

SA	A	U	D	SD
—	6%	3%	60%	31%

47. Most of the consultants seem to treat the other doctors who work for them as fairly equal members of the team.

SA	A	U	D	SD
6%	73%	10%	10%	1%

48. In this hospital many forms and other returns that do not deal with the patient are superfluous.

SA	A	U	D	SD
10%	32%	28%	29%	1%

49. It is no longer necessary to insist upon the ward staff using formal titles when working together.

SA	A	U	D	SD
3%	10%	4%	59%	24%

50. The best sister is often the most unpopular.

SA	A	U	D	SD
4%	19%	9%	47%	20%

51. Even in a ward with two or more consultants, sister should always deal with them herself.

SA	A	U	D	SD
7%	39%	8%	41%	5%

52. It does not matter what a nurse is thinking and feeling provided she is getting on with her work.

SA	A	U	D	SD
1%	8%	5%	63%	23%

53. There are times when the sister should be the first to point out that a mistake on her part has created misunderstanding.

SA	A	U	D	SD
30%	67%	1%	1%	1%

54. A sister at this hospital would be personally consulted about any proposals affecting her ward, whether coming from matron, the medical staff, the secretary, the engineer or any other quarter.

SA	A	U	D	SD
24%	51%	8%	14%	3%

55. Ward activity must be regulated for the medical staff's convenience.

SA	A	U	D	SD
6%	17%	9%	47%	21%

56. A sister who demands a high standard of work from her staff usually makes herself disliked by them.

SA	A	U	D	SD
3%	12%	7%	58%	20%

57. The hospital situation requires that new instructions should be issued in writing rather than by word of mouth.

SA	A	U	D	SD
15%	59%	11%	14%	1%

58. The consultants at this hospital all have their little ways of liking their prestige to be acknowledged.

SA	A	U	D	SD
10%	57%	17%	14%	2%

59. From time to time sister may need openly to question the traditional policies of the hospital.

SA	A	U	D	SD
8%	61%	18%	12%	1%

60. The medical staff should be more cooperative in choosing times for their ward visits.

SA	A	U	D	SD
29%	48%	7%	15%	—

61. Sisters need not attempt to explain to their subordinates instructions coming down from a higher level.

SA	A	U	D	SD
1%	16%	7%	57%	19%

62. Junior nurses should learn about the patient from sister rather than from the medical staff.

SA	A	U	D	SD
21%	54%	10%	14%	1%

63. The hospital cannot run smoothly unless sister believes that the senior staff are always right.

SA	A	U	D	SD
5%	18%	13%	53%	11%

64. Student nurses should be taught not to speak to the doctor unless spoken to first.

SA	A	U	D	SD
5%	29%	13%	45%	7%

65. If junior nurses have any complaints, they should make them through their ward sister.

SA	A	U	D	SD
23%	63%	6%	8%	—

66. The consultants here bring the junior medical staff into their important clinical decisions.

SA	A	U	D	SD
10%	64%	21%	4%	1%

Appendix 6
Sisters' attitudes as hospital characteristics

A note on the statistical significance of differences of attitudes between hospitals. (The data is not always drawn from the same samples as are referred to in chapter 7 and Appendix 5, but the results are typical.)

1. If we select as indicators of hierarchical commitment the sisters' responses to the three statements:

(a) in the planning the ward duty rota, preference for desirable hours and time off should be given according to seniority;

(b) the tradition that nursing staff of similar status should keep together at mealtimes is essential to the efficiency of the hospital; and

(c) one of the most important characteristics of a good nurse is the respect she shows for the medical staff,

we may accumulate the scores of these responses (as in Appendix 5, paragraph 3) and analyse the variance within and between hospitals. The results, for 350 sisters in 15 hospitals, are given in Table A6.1.

Table A6.1

Source of variation	Sum of squares	Degrees of freedom	Estimate of variance	F
Between hospitals	338	14	24·2	5·1
Within hospitals	1588	335	4·74	

For 14 and 335 degrees of freedom the 1 per cent and 0·1 per cent significance levels are about 2·2 and 2·8 respectively. There is thus no doubt that commitment to the opinions expressed in (a), (b) and (c) above is strongly associated with particular hospitals.

2. If we measure attitudes to the integration and training of student nurses by the responses of the sisters to the three following statements:

(d) most young people of today have had too soft an upbringing;

(e) education today gives the student nurse too much theory;
(f) sisters can devote time to instructing the student nurse only at the expense of what may be more important demands;

we may analyse the scores again as in paragraph 1 above. The results are set out in Table A6.2. (This result is for 352 ward sisters in 19 provincial acute general hospitals; this is a more homogeneous sample of hospitals than used to produce Table A6.1, which included teaching hospitals as well as ex-municipal infirmaries.)

Table A6.2

Source of variation	Sum of squares	Degrees of freedom	Estimate of variance	F
Between hospitals	304	18	16·9	2·77
Within hospitals	2038	333	6·1	

This result is significant at about 0·1 per cent, showing that attitudes towards training (as suggested by responses to items (d), (e) and (f)) differ much more between hospitals than they differ among the sisters within them.

3. If, finally, we measure the perception that ward sisters have of the organization for which they work by their responses to the following three statements (see Appendix 5):

(g) the matron and her administrative staff are no longer as closely in touch with ward problems as they should be;
(h) the medical staff tend to treat suggestions from nurses with less consideration than they deserve;
(i) ancillary departments, such as the pharmacy, kitchen or maintenance, seem to the sister to be organized for their own convenience rather than that of the wards;

Table A6.3

Source of variation	Sum of squares	Degrees of freedom	Estimate of variance	F
Between hospitals	264	18	14·7	2·53
Within hospitals	1925	333	5·8	

we may again analyse the scores as in paragraph 1. The results, for the same 352 sisters in the 19 hospitals referred to in paragraph 2, are given in Table A6.3.

This result is again significant at about 0·1 per cent, showing that perceptions of the organization itself differ much more between hospitals than they do among sisters in the same hospital.

4. These three results leave no doubt whatever of the existence of hospital characteristics. Whether we consider the mean commitments of sisters throughout any particular hospital to questions of status and seniority; or their sympathy towards student nurses; or their perceptions of the cooperativeness of those on whom they themselves depend in their own hospitals, there are highly significant differences between hospitals.

5. For the 19 hospitals referred to in paragraphs 2 and 3 above the coefficient of correlation between the 19 pairs of hospital means of:

(a) attitudes towards integration of student nurses and
(b) perceptions of cooperativensss of seniors

is + 0·601; this is highly significant (1 per cent = 0·561).

Hence senior staff in hospitals where ward sisters tend to display sympathetic attitudes toward student nurses seem in turn to display cooperative attitudes toward the ward sisters. There is, on the other hand, no correlation between pairs of hospital means involving status commitment as one of the two variates.

Appendix 7
Diagnostic group and social dependence

It was suggested in chapter 8 that hospital characteristics, as distinct from the personal skills of individual members of staff, are likely to influence, for better or for worse, the recovery rates of medical patients more than those of the surgical, since the medical patient is the more socially dependent, both for diagnosis and for treatment. It is said that the physician's trade demands that he be more socially aware and more dependent upon the ideas and suggestions of others than need be the more individualist surgeon. The physician seeks to interpret the signs that may first be noticed by others, the Joseph reading the Pharaoh's dream, the Daniel at the feast of Belshazzar; it is no coincidence that, whereas the assistant surgeon was known as the dresser, the assistant physician was known as the clerk. It would be interesting to examine the careers of successful doctor-administrators; according to this theory of social awareness and dependence one would expect comparatively few surgeons to succeed in the highly intuitive business of assessing human motive that is the chief preoccupation of the administrator.

However this may be, we may test the hypothesis of social dependence by examining the records of length of stay of medical and of surgical patients by hospitals. If we consider a set of medical patients in different diagnostic groups in the same hospital, and thus likely to be treated by different physicians, we should expect, if that hospital has a good communication system, all the medical patients, irrespective of diagnostic group, and hence of consultant, to recover more rapidly than they would in a hospital where the communication system was poor. All medical care, both in diagnosis and in treatment, in the one hospital would be more effective than all the medical care in the other hospital; there would, on the other hand, be a weaker 'hospital communication system influence', for good or ill, upon the surgical patients.

We show in Table A7.1 the mean lengths of stay of all the patients from 12 hospitals discharged home out of 12 diagnostic groups, six largely medical and six largely surgical. All hospitals are classified as acute or mainly acute; all are under the direction of the same Regional Board. The coefficient of concordance of the six medical groups is significantly greater than that of the six surgical. Since there are no known tests for comparing directly the significance of two such concordances, Table A7.2 sets out the arrays of rank order correlation coefficients, together with the sums of these coefficients set out against the diagnostic group, as giving some indication of the factor loadings. It is clear that

Rank orders by length of patient stay in six common medical and six common surgical diagnostic groups, for 12 acute general hospitals.

Hospital	Rank orders by length of patient stay											
	Medical cases						Surgical cases					
	OR	P	H	OD	AE	N	A	HR	O	MG	BN	FG
I	1	3	1	1	1	1	1	5	4	3	3½	10
II	2	2	7	4	4	2½	3	1	5	5	5	1
III	3	10	9	8	5	8	2	2	3	2	11	7½
IV	10	8	10	10	3	2½	6	10	2	11	2	2
V	5	1	3	2	7	6	10	6	6	8	9	6
VI	11	12	8	11	8	7	5	9	1	1	8	12
VII	4	7	4	5	2	5	9	7	8	9	12	3½
VIII	6	5	2	7	6	4	12	11	11	6	10	5
IX	9	4	6	3	10	10	8	4	9	4	3½	7½
X	7	6	5	9	9	12	4	3	7	7	1	3½
XI	12	11	11	12	11	9	7	12	12	12	6	11
XII	8	9	12	6	12	11	11	8	10	10	7	9

$$W = 0·56 \qquad\qquad W = 0·38$$

OR other respiratory diseases
P pneumonia
H diseases of heart
OD other diseases of digestive system
AE allergic and endocrine diseases, etc.
N diseases of central nervous system

A appendicitis
HR hernia of abdominal cavity
O diseases of bones and organs of locomotion
MG diseases of male genitals
BN Benign neoplasms
FG diseases of female genitals

these are significantly greater among the six medical groups. If the 30 correlation coefficients are transformed to Fisher's z, which is normally distributed, the difference between the means of the two sets of six sums is significant at 1 per cent.

Table A7.2
Rank order correlation coefficients of lengths of patient stay in 12 hospitals, by six medical and six surgical diagnostic groups.

	P	H	OD	AE	N	Sum		HR	O	MG	BN	FG	Sum
OR	61	58	70	67	49	3·05	A	57	66	52	38	−03	2·10
P		70	84	33	40	2·88	HR		33	52	14	33	1·89
H			63	50	53	2·84	O			52	11	08	1·70
OD				33	33	2·83	MG				−11	−29	1·16
AE					86	2·69	BN					15	0·67
N						2·51	FG						0·24

In the 30 correlation coefficients of these two arrays, all zeros and decimal points are omitted.

This therefore shows that, at least in these 12 (typical) hospitals there is a hospital influence, for good or ill, upon the progress of the medical patients significantly greater than upon the progress of the surgical. Hospital influences, of course, affect both classes; the surgeons also rely upon communications and upon the support of their nurses. But their dependence, although observable in Tables A7.1 and A7.2, is significantly less than is the dependence of the physicians.

Appendix 8
Duration of patient stay and relative mortality rates

1. A Regional Hospital Board produced a survey on 1 July, 1960 of the disposal of all patients at 14 general hospitals in its region. This survey classified all the patients at the hospitals by both diagnostic group and by disposal, either dead, discharged home, or transferred to another hospital or unit for further treatment or recovery; the data are for the year 1957. Since the survey was initiated, prepared, published and discussed without reference to this present study it may be regarded as an unbiased source of random information.

2. In using this survey to test the hypothesis that some hospital factor may influence the mean duration of patient stay, a factor independent of the disease treated, the data for 11 hospitals only were analysed. One was rejected because the number of cases in certain diagnostic groups was too small (less than 20); two more were rejected because of the high proportion of beds (42 per cent and 80 per cent) allocated to long-stay patients.

3. The five diagnostic groups accounting for the majority of hospital deaths were chosen for statistical study. They are:

(a) malignant neoplasms
(b) diseases of the central nervous system
(c) diseases of the heart
(d) pneumonia and
(e) other diseases of the digestive system.

Between them these five account for just over 70 per cent of all hospital deaths in the sample of 11 hospitals.

4. Table A8.1 sets out, by 11 rows and five columns, the mean duration of stay for all patients discharged home. The hospitals are placed roughly in rank order of duration, all five diagnostic groups being ranked separately and the hospital with the smallest sum of its rank orders appearing at the top. AA's rank orders are 2, 1, 1, 3, 1, total 8; LL's 11, 10, 11, 10, 11, total 53. It can be shown that there is a tendency, as apparent in these two hospitals, for rank orders to keep in step; the coefficient of concordance, W, is 0·60 and so high a value as this could have occurred by chance only once in a thousand times. Since we found it at our first attempt it is difficult to believe that it was a random result of sampling. We must assume, on the contrary, that there is a cause tending to influence the dura-

Table A8.1

Mean length of stay in days for all patients discharged home in five diagnostic groups, for 11 general hospitals in one region.

Hospital	Malig. neo.	CNS	Heart	Pneumonia	Digest. syst.
AA	21·8	16·4	18·6	15·2	13·8
BB	18·6	17·5	29·0	14·8	15·7
CC	24·4	17·9	25·0	14·2	14·7
DD	24·8	17·7	20·9	16·4	17·2
EE	26·2	17·8	24·2	17·1	16·6
FF	26·6	32·2	27·6	15·9	15·3
GG	23·8	18·9	26·5	16·8	18·4
HH	23·9	17·5	30·8	18·1	19·8
JJ	22·6	19·6	29·2	25·4	19·9
KK	25·7	21·2	30·3	21·9	18·3
LL	33·5	24·7	33·2	22·8	20·6

Source: a Regional Hospital Board's Statistics.

tion of stay at any hospital, whatever the disease for which the patient is under treatment at that hospital.

5. It is true that the percentages of beds occupied by long-stay patients varies between hospitals. Table A8.2 presents the figures; these show, for example, that AA has no long-stay patients, whereas LL had 25 per cent, or 31 beds out of 124. We have therefore divided the 11 hospitals into two classes; the first four form class S, with 156 beds out of 1670 occupied by long-stay patients, while the remaining seven hospitals form class L with 97 long-stay beds out of 1586. Class S hospitals thus have significantly more long-stay beds among them; all are in the same hospital, CC.

6. Table A8.2 also shows the disposal of the patients in these five diagnostic groups. Consider first the transfers to other hospitals or to convalescent units; in all five diagnostic groups the ratio of patients transferred to patients discharged home is greater in class L than in class S. The difference is not always significant, but it is always in favour of class L. It cannot be argued, therefore, that the four hospitals of class S, taken together, had the consistently shorter durations because they had easier access to discharge by transfer than had the seven hospitals of class L.

7. Table A8.2 also shows the relation between the numbers of deaths and of discharges home in each class by each diagnostic group. In two groups, diseases of the central nervous system and pneumonia, class L has a significantly larger number of deaths than class S; in the three other diagnostic groups there is no difference between the two classes of hospital. There is thus no evidence to suggest that the hospitals of class S, with the significantly shorter stay of patients discharged home, has a higher incidence of deaths per 100 admissions. We are

Table A8.2

Total number of beds, and of beds occupied by long-stay cases, 1957 (a); and numbers of patients in five diagnostic groups who, in that year, died (b); were discharged home (c); and who were transferred to another hospital (d), for 11 general hospitals in one region.

Hospital	Total	Long-stay beds (a) no.	Long-stay beds (a) %	Malignant neo. (b)	Malignant neo. (c)	Malignant neo. (d)	Dis. of CNS (b)	Dis. of CNS (c)	Dis. of CNS (d)	Dis. of heart (b)	Dis. of heart (c)	Dis. of heart (d)	Pneumonia (b)	Pneumonia (c)	Pneumonia (d)	Other Dis. of DS (b)	Other Dis. of DS (c)	Other Dis. of DS (d)
AA	109	—	—	25	56	9	21	35	—	10	26	1	7	42	1	13	80	2
BB	263	—	—	69	220	26	50	123	11	90	164	6	42	107	4	18	315	6
CC	608	156	26	113	311	23	81	205	27	101	246	7	32	388	6	16	481	10
DD	690	—	—	231	538	71	127	278	99	163	441	59	114	688	33	55	701	14
Totals Class S	1670	156	9	438	1125	129	279	641	137	364	877	73	195	1225	44	102	1577	32
EE	365	—	—	85	331	59	62	122	26	68	185	42	44	127	13	23	270	47
FF	198	14	7	30	94	24	21	39	10	22	47	10	18	78	5	4	98	6
GG	410	37	9	65	118	14	83	99	28	74	133	12	52	118	15	14	148	6
HH	147	—	—	45	153	41	31	35	12	27	49	8	12	46	8	6	129	35
JJ	190	15	8	30	87	22	23	47	7	28	54	9	5	30	5	9	146	16
KK	152	—	—	31	53	1	23	20	3	15	53	4	4	26	2	7	141	5
LL	124	31	25	44	55	5	22	34	7	28	53	6	11	28	2	6	71	2
Totals Class L	1586	97	6	330	891	166	265	396	93	262	574	91	146	453	50	69	1003	117

dealing here with very large numbers of patients, although it would be interesting to see this analysis for a larger sample of hospitals. For the present, however, the general argument that hospitals which discharge patients home rapidly may in some way be scamping their duty to the patient finds no evidence in the mortality rates of otherwise comparable hospitals. It is, of course, argued throughout this book that, provided the short stay is a *consequence* of that efficiency which derives from good communications, then there is no harm, indeed, every likelihood of benefit, to the patient treated in the hospital which discharged sooner rather than later. Suggestions that one hospital whose mean duration of stay is up to one week less than that of another (comparing like with like) is in some way necessarily depriving its patients of better service do not find support in the evidence, if that service is to be measured by the probability of dying in hospital from one of the five major killing diseases.

Bibliography

Books

Barnes, E., *People in Hospital*, Macmillan, London, 1961.
Bevington, S., *Nursing Life and Discipline*, London, 1943.
Cartwright, A., *Human Relations and Hospital Care*, Institute of Community Studies, 1963.
Lindsey, A., *Socialised Medicine in England and Wales—National Health Service 1948/61*, Oxford University Press, 1962.
McGhee, A., *The Patient's Attitude to Nursing Care*, Livingstone, Edinburgh, 1961.
Smith, B. A., *A History of the Nursing Profession*, Heinemann, 1960.
Woodham-Smith, C., *Florence Nightingale*, Constable, London, 1950.

Reports and periodicals

Action Society Trust papers, 1955–9:
  1. *Background and Blueprint*
  2. *The Impact of Change*
  3. *Groups, Regions and Committees, Part 1*, HMC
  4. *Part II, Regional Hospital Boards*
  5. *Central Control of the Services*
  6. *Creative Leadership in a State Service*
Barr, A., 'The training of student nurses', *British Journal of Social and Preventive Medicine*, **13**, 3, 1959.
Barr, A., H. M. V. Smith and L. James, *Some Results of Training Student Nurses in General Hospitals*, Monthly Bulletin of the Ministry of Health, 1957.
Beveridge, W., *Social Insurance and Allied Services*, (Beveridge Report), Macmillan, London, 1942.
Bradbeer Report, *Internal Administration of Hospitals*, Central Health Services Council, HMSO, London, 1953.
Chambers, V. E., 'Hospital cadet schemes and their impact on the recruitment and training of nurses in the Manchester region', unpublished Ph.D. thesis, 1960.
Cohen Report, *Minority Report*, HMSO, London, 1948.

Crichton, A., *Report on a Survey—Administrative and Clerical Staffs in Hospitals in Wales, 1960–1961*, Welsh Regional Hospital Board.

Cross, K. S., and D. L. A. Hall, 'Survey of entrants to nurse training schools and of student nurse wastage in the Birmingham region', *British Journal of Social and Preventive Medicine*, **8,** 1954.

General Nursing Council for England and Wales: Annual Report to the Ministry of Health, 1959 to 1962.

Guillebaud Report, *Report of the Committee of Inquiry into the Cost of the National Health Service*, HMSO, London, 1956.

Lancet Commission on Nursing, *Lancet*, London, 1932.

Maguire, J., *From Student to Nurse*, Oxford Regional Hospital Board, 1961.

Dan Mason Research Committee, National Florence Nightingale Committee of Great Britain and Northern Ireland, *The Work of Recently Qualified Nurses*, London, 1956.

Dan Mason Research Committee, National Florence Nightingale Committee of Great Britain and Northern Ireland, *The Work of Student Nurses and Pupil Assistant Nurses*, London, July 1957.

Dan Mason Research Committee, National Florence Nightingale Committee of Great Britain and Northern Ireland, *The Work, Responsibilities and Status of the Enrolled Nurse*, London, 1962.

Menzies, I., 'A case study of the functioning of social systems as a defence against anxiety', *Human Relations*, **13,** 2, 1960.

Ministry of Health, *Inter-departmental Committee on Nursing Services: Interim Report (Athlone Committee),* HMSO, London, 1939.

Noel Hall Report, *Report on the Grading Structure of Administrative and Clerical Staff in the Hospital Service*, HMSO, London, 1957.

Nuffield Provincial Hospitals Trust, *The Work of Nurses in Hospital Wards—Report of a Job Analysis*, London, 1953.

The Pattern of the In-Patient's Day, Central Health Services Council, HMSO, London, 1961.

Platt Report, *Report of the Joint Working Party on the Medical Staffing Structures in the Hospital Service*, HMSO, London, 1960.

Porritt Report, *A Review of Medical Services in Great Britain*, Medical Services Review Committee, London, 1962.

Report of the Ministry of Health for the year ended 31st December, 1958. Parts I and II, (and subsequently to December, 1962), HMSO.

Report of the Working Party on Recruitment and Training of Nurses, Ministry of Health, Department of Health for Scotland and Ministry of Labour and National Service, HMSO, London, 1947.

Revans, R. W., *The Hospital as an Organism,* Proceedings of the 6th International Meeting of the Institute of Management Sciences, Pergamon Press, London, 1960.

Revans, R. W., *The Measurement of Supervisory Attitudes*, Manchester Statistical Society, January, 1961.

Revans, R. W., 'Hospitals attitudes and communications', *Sociological Review Monograph*, July, 1962.

Royal College of Nursing—Observations and Objectives, London, 1956.

Seeman, M., and J. W. Evans, 'Stratification and hospital care II—The objective criteria of performance', *American Sociological Review*, **26,** 2, April, 1961.

Srivastava, M. P., 'The morale of hospital nurses—a study of wastage and sickness in the Manchester region', unpublished Ph.D. thesis.

Wallis, K. F., 'Length of patient stay in hospitals—an analytical study', unpublished M.Sc. thesis.

Woodward, J., *Employment Relations in a Group of Hospitals*, Institute of Hospital Administration, London, 1950.

PART TWO

The Hospitals' Internal Communications Project
by Janet B. Craig

Introduction

This part of our book describes some efforts to follow up the suggestions of chapter 9 of Part One, *Standards for Morale*: 'The hospitals themselves, personified by their administrators, their doctors and their nurses . . . must learn to conduct surveys, to interpret their findings, to seek the structure of the problems so revealed, and to build the programmes of participation by which those problems may be ameliorated.' Hospital staffs were urged to diagnose their own organizational problems and to seek appropriate therapy from their own resources; this would demand much more self-awareness and self-disclosure than was traditional in some hospitals, where the need was for staff to perceive the effects that individuals had upon each other and upon the hospital as a whole. The exercises that followed are described as a series of action learning projects, each following upon and gaining from its predecessors. We do not propose to go once more into the operational details of these separate endeavours; there are adequate accounts of them in other references (see References, Part Two, pages 149 and 155). Our concern now is with the launching of the whole enterprise, and with what needed to be done between the first proposals for self-diagnosis and for autotherapy set forth in *Standards for Morale*, on the one hand, and on the other, getting something done about those proposals on the wards and in the operating theatres of a few real hospitals. Although it is a principle of action learning that one judges any system only by its output, any endeavour only by what it achieves, any person only by his deeds, it is nonetheless interesting to record how the processes of diagnosis and therapy were actually got going: what they succeeded in doing has been described elsewhere, particularly in Part Three of this work, *An evaluation of the HIC Project*. In the present part we devote most of our attention to this project, since its novelty at the time caused so much comment, both sympathetic and hostile, and because so many other exercises, alike in hospitals and elsewhere, have grown from it.

10. Theory into practice

The stresses of integration

Standards for Morale is said to have become a textbook for students of hospital administration because the lessons learned in the Lancashire hospitals in 1964 remain relevant to hospital life today. Moreover, not only must hospital staff learn to communicate more effectively for the good of the patient: staff throughout the health service, both inside and out of hospital, are expected, since April 1974, to unify the service by closer cooperation. Learning must now bring not only different persons into a better mutual understanding: it must encourage cooperation between institutions that were previously remote and not seldom in competition. The need for autonomous learning has suddenly taken on a deeper significance. How then was this need seen when the suggestion to do something about it was first put forward? In February 1964, when *Standards for Morale* was published, widely read and discussed, the argument centred mainly around the validity or otherwise of one research finding, that mean length of patient stay was related to staff morale. Did this mean that the real message—let the hospitals examine their own actions and we will help them—was not understood? Or was it so clearly understood that it was safe to ignore it?

Some supposed maladies had been diagnosed in hospitals in the Manchester area. In 1965, after a year's prompting by King Edward's Hospital Fund for London, some London hospitals accepted the challenge to find the therapy, and the Ministry of Health agreed to finance a project in their support. It had first been necessary to show that a reasonable number of hospitals were willing to undertake the study before the Ministry were prepared to give financial backing as a three-year research grant, and to understand the task undertaken by Revans and the King's Fund in getting ten London hospitals to volunteer for the study, one needs to know something of the Health Service at that time.

Unlike the 1976 Department of Health and Social Security, the 1964 Ministry of Health divided the provision for the nation's health between different services, the three main being general practice, the local authority and the hospital. The hospital service had regional and teaching hospital boards to control how hospitals should be managed, although at that time much of their thought and income were taken in designing and building large district general hospitals to replace many small and specialist hospitals. In preparation for these all-purpose hospitals, the existing hospitals were grouped and run by hospital group secretaries, group medical committees and group matrons. It was a troublesome time for hospital staff; they had lost the chiefs they were used to and were suspicious of new faces in new offices; some secretaries and matrons had been chiefs and now they had someone to whom they had to answer. Schools of nursing of long standing and good repute were having to join forces with less eminent ones in group nursing schools, arousing again uncomfortable feelings of lost prestige.

Inside individual hospitals in 1964, changes had been developing painfully and slowly since the introduction of the Health Service in 1948.[1] There was not much sign of nurse, doctor and other staff working as a team; each seemed to follow their independent line towards their own perception of what was good for the patient. Most matrons had yielded up some of their responsibilities for services, often with reluctance, especially if the services were critical for the comfort and welfare of the patients. Arguments were still frequent between matrons and secretaries about such issues as the supply and shortage of clean linen, or to whom the domestic superintendent should be responsible. In the wards, staff and patients were affected by the same worries as the matrons and secretaries; linen and cleanliness of the wards were their problems, too. They also shared with their seniors the problems of the shorter working week, and of increased tuition for student nurses in the school and away from the wards. They had more nurses—on paper—but fewer, in fact, to care for the greater number of patients being admitted and discharged each day. What was forcing the change, more quickly than the new administration of the health service itself, upon doctors, nurses and patients at ward level, was the rapid growth of medical science and technology. The junior doctors and the nurses, whether handling the machines or treating the patients, were gaining more knowledge about disease and its cure than were the senior staff more absorbed in routine procedures and administration. In hospital conditions such as are described in *Standards for Morale*, where all communication is downwards, the frustrations which the pressures of this new knowledge at lower levels caused can well be imagined.

The Manchester Regional Hospital Board and the Nuffield Provincial Hospitals Trust must be congratulated in seeing the need, already in the mid-fifties, to examine the organizational problems of hospitals in the region. They can have had little idea as to how far-reaching their decision would be. Nowadays most senior hospital personnel are conscious of the need for management skills; many have shared in participative management exercises, in which members of different disciplines pool their skills, knowledge and other resources in better ways to manage the critical situations which so often arise. Multi-disciplinary meetings, conferences and seminars are now common. In 1964, however, few doctors or nurses thought of themselves as managers. The most they would accept was to manage their own sphere only. The idea of working together was new; it threatened deep historical, hierarchical and inter-disciplinary barriers, and generated yet more anxiety in the exercise of their now crumbling but once authoritarian hospital routines. This then was the prevailing climate in which the King's Fund invited Revans to attempt some therapy with the ten London hospitals who recognized in themselves the maladies he had diagnosed in the Manchester region. We know of no earlier meeting where doctors, nurses and administrators, as a congress of teams from differing hospitals, were invited to meet together to exhibit their common problems and to decide upon methods of attempting to solve them.

The selection of hospitals

In the spring of 1964 Revans, after two or three discussions and much correspondence, was invited by the King's Fund Centre to offer some of the hospitals in London the opportunity of studying their own internal communication systems with a view to improving their own efficiency. Quite how the hospitals should undertake the study could not at that time be explained; much was to depend upon the senior staff of the hospitals concerned as to how committed they allowed themselves and other staff working with them to become.

The problem of which hospitals out of the 500 or so in London to invite to join the project was overcome in the early summer of 1964, when the King's Fund gave the four Metropolitan Regional Hospital Board secretaries the opportunity of meeting with Revans. The advice of these very senior health service staff was sought as to how the hospitals should be selected. The secretaries were hesitant about recommending the project to hospitals in their regions but finally decided to seek volunteers through each of the next regional meetings for hospital group secretaries. They were asked to offer this opportunity to, at the most, six hospitals in each region. It was the end of September 1964 before all four regional boards had held their meetings of hospital group secretaries, and before lists of hospitals willing to be invited to hear more of the proposed study began to come into the Centre. The letter of invitation sent by return to each nominee mentioned the date of a meeting with Revans and asked the group secretary to bring with him senior medical and nursing staff. Altogether about two dozen group secretaries and chief administrators of London teaching hospitals accepted the invitation to attend this November meeting, bringing with them a medical consultant and the matron of a hospital or her deputy.

The meeting was chaired by Sir Robert Platt (now Lord Platt) who warmly recommended the type of study envisaged. Revans then spoke of a paper previously circulated and invited the hospital staff to comment on his proposals. The suggestion that poor morale was a consequence of (among other things) inadequate administration, just as much in the hospitals of London today as it had been in the coal mines before nationalization and in the Manchester hospitals since they had been nationalized, aroused vigorous expressions of emotion. People spoke angrily from the floor and rejected outright the request to release members of staff for six months to learn the methods they might need to examine the effectiveness of their own management. Just as strongly opposed was another recommendation that staff from one hospital should be on such terms with staff from another hospital that members of peer groups might call each other in to help solve a problem defying those on the spot. Medical consultants

119

spoke of their time being fully occupied in treating the illnesses of their patients, leaving them no freedom to share in solving problems of patient comfort and well-being while in hospital. The nurses expressed the view that the welfare of patients was their concern and not that of others working in the hospital remote from the bedside.

It was anticipated that not all the hospitals represented at this first meeting would continue to display interest in the proposal. Those who were prepared to negotiate further were invited to another meeting in December 1964. The key to the success of this meeting was the realization that having rejected most of Revans' proposals at the first meeting, the hospital staff now had the opportunity—indeed, the obligation—to put forward their own proposals.

A project was suggested which would involve a mixed group of staff in examining their services to the patients. But whatever design was explored, nobody seemed able to find time to work on it. No member of staff could be spared for six or even three months for a course. Neither could they be spared one day or half a day once each week. How much time would have to be given to the project once the learners were back in post? Revans' suggestion, that one-third of their time should be devoted to using the methods learned on the course, was alarming. His explanation that the project would be involving people during their normal work, even if doing it differently, went unheeded. By the end of this second meeting the hospital staff found themselves agreeing to continue to explore the possibilities of a project. Perhaps they could spare themselves, the top people, for a three-day residential course to learn how to support the less senior doctors, nurses and administrators once they returned; having gained the rudiments of research techniques, at a one-month course. In sharing these experiences, perhaps, the teams would become able to support each other once back in their own hospitals. At least two years would be needed for the hospital teams to complete any worthwhile project within their own hospitals. Encouraged by these cautious admissions, Revans spoke of the isolation of hospitals and their need to exchange impressions with other organizations (as he then believed), particularly with universities. He said he would like the teams to become proficient in explaining their studies not only to their peers, but also the world outside. For them to gain practice in this he suggested regular seminars, three or four a year, in some academic setting where the teams could present their studies to an audience interested in the social sciences and the functioning of organizations.

After each large meeting for hospital staff, those responsible for the conduct of the meetings and one or two others sat down to discuss their impressions of how the hospitals were responding and what next step should be taken. Staff from the Research Department of the Ministry of Health attended the main meetings and afterwards joined the group discussions. In December 1964 they were sufficiently confident to promise—provided enough hospitals volunteered to join the project taking shape—that the Ministry would provide £5000 in the first instance. When asked by the King's Fund to give a definite answer by the end of 1964 as to whether they were willing to join in a three-year project, the hospitals were unprepared. Besides the lack of time allowed for making such a decision, other reasons for withdrawal were discovered. Some did not understand the object of this study and others doubted its methods; a few representatives lacked the support of their management committees, and one group could not see that they needed any self-examination at all. By January 1965, however, the King's Fund was able to tell the Ministry that eight hospitals had accepted the opportunity offered and others were still considering the proposition. Eight hospitals were sufficient to secure the initial allocation of money. In the end ten hospitals joined the consortium.

Advice, evaluation, and control

In January, 1965 a director of the project was appointed. After a very short time he had a small team of people who, if they had not worked with Revans, at least claimed to be familiar with the approach he was developing and interested to help. This group of people became known as the central team, which fluctuated in size throughout the three years of the study. Their task, as seen by the King's Fund, was to prepare and conduct the initial study courses for the hospital staff, to convene the inter-hospital and academic meetings and to act as a resource to whom the hospital teams could refer for help in their own local exercises. The novelty of the approach demanded such tutelage, for not only was the intermingling of diversified hospital staff from different hospitals a new experience for them, for the research workers, too, it was unknown to assist staff in examining their own work instead of examining it for them. Those supporting the project were equally unfamiliar with the art of monitoring rather than directing the several projects which were to be attempted. It was as if all were trying to prevent others from hurting themselves.

To add to the necessary complexities of the project a team was brought in to evaluate the project. This team had to work alongside the central team in the same already overcrowded office and attempt an independent piece of work; they became auditors who could hear all and see all, but who were permitted to contribute nothing in return. Some tension between the dozen teams was therefore not unexpected.

It was, moreover, not the custom for the Ministry of Health and Social Security to hold the monies for any research it was backing. The King's Fund were also reluctant to undertake this custodial task. It was also recognized that the project would gain status if it could be brought under the general guidance of some university department. Guy's Medical School agreed to elect Revans a research fellow, to hold the project accounts and, through their department of community medicine, to assume responsibility for the studies done in the cooperating hospitals. Thus, two members of staff from the King's Fund, as the instigators, two from the research department of the Ministry, as the backers, and two from the Department of Community Medicine, as the research agents, found themselves forming a steering committee to monitor the project as it developed.

The steering committee was divided throughout the project in their perceptions of the relative emphasis to put on the involvement of hospital staff in formulating and conducting their own studies, on the one hand, and, on the other, the sociological and other pure research to be undertaken by the central and evaluating teams. The King's Fund favoured the first, in the main, carrying the hospitals with them. But the Ministry or, as it eventually became, the Department of Health and Social Security, favoured the second. Guy's Medical School accepted the role of mediator throughout the three years, although they were naturally influenced by both the source of the money and by their responsibilities to the research teams. Revans had envisioned the hospitals being involved in examining themselves, and had also seen the research workers (besides acting as resource people) learning for themselves through this novel experience, producing papers for professional journals and, perhaps, theses for higher degrees. He had anticipated joint problem solving, in which all would be learning to their own advantage and the good of the whole. Others could not believe that unqualified staff could undertake proper research. Yet learning there was, although painfully achieved. Harmony there was not, rather a deep division in outlook where help given to one side was seen as neglect to the other. It is said the attitude of those at the top of any organization has a great influence upon those beneath, starting a chain reaction from the top down. The divisions in the steering committee must have contributed to the tensions which arose between themselves, the other groups of central and evaluation teams, and hospital staff. Tension mounted throughout the project, between and within these four interests. Like the hospitals it hoped to help, the project itself was cradled in anxiety; moreover these internal struggles could convey a false impression of the project and might lead future initiators unawares into no less painful a situation. Those of us who are still struggling to judge our own original efforts in the study have now learned that all exercises in action learning are likely to expose profound differences in values, aims and aspirations among the people involved. Instead of attempting, as we did in this original project, to impose our own specific aims (namely, hospital learning by hospital doing) upon everyone else, we now have seen the wisdom of multi-disciplinary teams progressively evolving a multi-purpose exercise. This, besides giving individual satisfaction, adds to the richness of the findings and the significance of the action taken as a result.

The choice of hospital teams

As we have seen, the regional hospital board secretaries asked hospital group secretaries to volunteer their hospitals' involvement in the communications project. This the group secretaries did with varying amounts of backing from their hospital management committees. Support ranged from passive consent, through the hospital staff helping to design exercises, as far as actual involvement of committee members themselves. The group secretaries each invited their matron and a medical or surgical consultant to join them at the King's Fund meetings, to develop with Revans some plan of specific action. These three from each hospital became the senior hospital team ready to attend the three-day course for senior staff. One of the first tasks of this senior team was to ensure that its hospital appointed a junior or operational study team to arrange the field surveys and any corrective action these surveys might suggest.

Who then selected, how did they select and for what motives, those members of hospital staff who eventually formed the junior hospital teams? This has never been fully explained or explored. Many of the team members from the same hospital met for the first time, as strangers, on the project and had great difficulty in understanding not only why they had been chosen to come but what was expected of them. The most representative junior hospital team comprised a hospital secretary, an assistant matron and either a medical or surgical consultant. Sometimes the nurse was a senior ward sister. The medical member of the junior team was the most elusive to recruit. Registrars were most generally considered to be ideal, but somehow they were too busy preparing clinical research material or afraid of losing their chance of promotion by having their attention diverted from clinical work, to what was regarded as mere administration.

Those responsible for launching the project were conscious of the difficult task, and the selection of a final team was left to the hospital group secretary. All sorts of reasons (soon to become all too familiar) were given for not being able to form a team: lack of staff; lack of time; too much research already; too much involvement in change; transfer of the hospital to new buildings. All these were seen as more urgent than learning about the present style of communications and how these affect the care of the patient.

11. Field activities

In May, 1965, the project was launched with the three-day course for the senior hospital staff, namely, the group secretary, the group matron and a medical or surgical consultant from each of the ten hospitals. They were encouraged by the presence of the Minister of Health, Mr Kenneth Robinson, in person, and by the discourses of visitors from Denmark and the USA, expert in organizational change and the value of staff involvement. The senior staff left knowing that somehow they had to find a junior hospital team to attend the month's residential course in 1965. This gave doctors, nurses and administrators the opportunities promised. They learned some research techniques and became able to discuss freely their hospital problems with colleagues from other hospitals. Perhaps what they had feared most, but later claimed as the most useful part of their four weeks, was the third week they spent in each others' hospitals looking into and reporting upon problems of their own choosing.

Once back in their own hospitals, over the next two years, the junior hospital teams, with varying amounts of assistance from their senior colleagues, set about their own studies. The central team monitored what was happening and gave help when asked for and where they saw the need. The evaluation team, having arrived after the training courses were over, started by picking up impressions of what had already been achieved, then designed and eventually used their methods of measurement. Besides going into individual hospitals, the central team organized inter-hospital meetings at the King's Fund Centre and less frequently at the London School of Hygiene and Tropical Medicine. The former were for hospital teams to compare progress and the latter to give one hospital at a time the opportunity of explaining its study to a wider audience.

The steering committee seemed to meet only at the suggestion of the central team. News of individual hospital studies was received second hand through the central and evaluation teams. On one occasion nearing the end of the project the hospitals did manage to meet the steering committee, but only to find themselves 'talked at' and not given the opportunity to discuss problems relating to the project as a whole. The necessity of those steering a project to be as involved and as approachable as those undertaking field work is another lesson learned from this essentially cooperative project.

Yet one more example of the divisions within and between the many interests involved in the study became evident over the publication of the findings. There were those who thought one publication written by the research teams, a supposedly scientific report, alone was needed. Others felt if there was only to be one book then it should be written by the hospital staffs involved in the studies. There were others again who recommended both should be published together. In the end two books were published but separately, the scientific research treatise first and the hospitals' account three or four months later. Whereas the project had favourable notice in the technical press at the outset, the book reviews in the same journals some years later were not favourable, and some critics condemned the basic idea of hospital staff involvement as an imbecility, even if well intended. Just as Revans' original recommendations for autotherapy in *Standards for Morale* went largely unnoticed, so the innovatory notions of autonomous group learning developed in this project made no impression in the world of administrative or organizational science—at that time.

Individual hospital studies

Readers are referred to the full accounts of all the hospital studies written by the hospital staff. These can be found in *Hospitals: Communications, Choice and Change*.[1] Of the ten contributions in that book, four are set out in this chapter:

Hillingdon Hospital
Lewisham Hospital
The London Hospital
North Middlesex Hospital

These in particular have been chosen as examples of the variable quality and quantity of learning which took place. Some hospitals found that the study of one problem led to another; a greater number of people were in this way involved in looking at themselves. This led to a general sense of institutional awareness developing throughout some of the ten hospitals. In contrast, however, some hospital teams could see no purpose in the project, involved no more staff and found other work too pressing to allow them to attempt any further study. (Later researches, flowing directly from the project but conducted at the Southern Methodist University, Dallas, Texas, suggest that about a third of the population has been immunized by earlier education against learning from its own experience. See also Part Three.)

Hillingdon Hospital by Marie Perkins

Hillingdon Hospital participants

W. E. Bardgett*	group secretary
G. W. Duncan*	medical administrator
R. Dunkley**	deputy group secretary
J. A. Monro**	consultant anaesthetist
Marie Perkins**	deputy matron
Eleanor Roker*	matron

* Attended three-day appreciation course, 1965.
** Attended one-month course, 1965.

This hospital, about 15 miles west of London, has 772 beds and serves over a quarter of a million people. Over 14 000 in-patients and about 185 000 out-patients are cared for each year.

The hospital offers general nurse training for state registration (three years), state enrolment (two years), and full training courses for midwifery, health visiting, and district nursing. There are also postgraduate courses in out-patient and casualty work, operating theatre and the nursing of premature babies, and a pre-nursing course for cadet nurses, in conjunction with a polytechnic course in further education.

In October 1965 I found myself seconded to the HIC training course as the operational-nurse member, with the administrative and medical members. The course proved of value. Much was to be learned and gained by the interchanging of ideas, discussing and recognizing the other man and his problems, seeing that problems so often are common to many of us, and that the solving of them can be approached from different angles. The theme throughout seemed to be lack of communication, and the manner in which communications were handled. The complexity of this manifested itself the more the subject was analysed. The need to do a simple task thoroughly to avoid complication became evident, as did the importance of understanding why a thing does or does not work, and of discovering whether improvements can be made in its operation. The tools required for any job must be provided. The techniques and skills were taught and put into practice during the third week of the course, which was spent working in one of the other hospitals represented on the course. This in itself stressed the need for working as a whole team and not as isolated units, just as the patient needs to be treated as a human being, a complete whole.

The hospital opened a large new building in January 1967. To some extent, preparing for this prevented our team from embarking on projects in which we could apply the skills and techniques taught on the course. The demand emerged as the new building gradually became fully operational.[2]

The first matter needing attention at this stage seemed to be the messenger service. This was investigated and improved by only minor alterations. The fact that the new wing produced certain geographical changes proved to be an asset. New buildings produce new blood, new ideas; change is not acceptable to all but is essential to the well-being of the patient.

Increases in recruitment of nursing staff in all grades, resident and non-resident, produced complications with regard to duty rotas and transport, partly through lack of resident accommodation. These problems were considered and found to offer an opportunity to try out recently acquired skills and techniques. The central team helped by carrying out an attitude survey among the nursing staff. A questionnaire was drawn up and sent out to 470 nursing staff. A psychology student joined us to help define workloads on the wards and the basic and technical nursing hours required over a 24-hour period.

This project gave us an opportunity to introduce some new methods of communication, in particular group discussions.

It is planned in future to use the skills of the operational team to solve ap-

126

propriate problems as they arise, rather than to search out possible projects when other matters (not necessarily for the team to solve) may be more pressing.

Briefly, the fact that more staff have been given the opportunity to express their views by use of questionnaires, meetings, free interviews, and the like, has resulted in a feeling of belonging rather more closely, instead of learning and direction by remote control. The community has now realized that snap decisions are not made, that discussion takes place, and that major projects and procedures are not the brain-child of one individual, which seemed at one time to be the belief of some of the staff. Complacency seems to have given away to alertness, and dissatisfaction seems to have lessened.

Additional comments by W. E. Bardgett

My own view, for what it is worth, is that the HIC Project suffered from too much pressure to produce results by its techniques, when in the hospitals there may have been more pressing problems which had to be solved by other methods. This, I believe, was the case at our hospital where, during most of the Project period, we were concerned with the overriding task of completing, equipping, moving into, and commissioning the new hospital building. It is only since the move has been completed that we have begun to use HIC techniques to solve a real problem, the one concerning nursing staff described by my colleague.

This criticism of the HIC Project draws attention to a fundamental problem about the way in which the project was financed and the research workers concerned with it were employed. If they had formed part of the permanent staff of a regional board or other hospital authority, or of the Ministry itself, it would have been possible to use their services as appropriate problems arose and there would have been less pressure to demonstrate the value of HIC techniques during a limited research period and, presumably, in order to ensure that research grants were renewed. This, I think, gave rise to requests and pressures to use the techniques which eventually became irritating to those at hospital level, particularly where, as in our own case, those concerned were overwhelmingly preoccupied with other matters.

One further criticism I have to make, with the benefit of hindsight, is that there was a lack of definition of the purpose at the Hastings course. It seemed to be a collection of interesting lectures with an insufficient central theme. I believe that the hospital people on the course could have contributed more by cooperating with the research workers in devising ways in which communication in hospitals might be improved, and I think too much emphasis was placed upon demonstrating the connections between poor communications and other shortcomings, at the expense of not devoting sufficient time to devising practical means of improving matters.

Lewisham Hospital by Marjorie Bell and A. J. Brooking

Lewisham Hospital participants

Marjorie Bell*	matron
A. J. Brooking*	group secretary

* Attended three-day appreciation course, 1965.

127

R. C. Cains**	administrator‡
A. Cavendish**	consultant surgeon
B. E. W. Mace*	consultant in physical medicine
J. W. Thompson†	hospital secretary (replaced R. C. Cains)
Grace White**	ward sister

and departmental heads and ward sisters of Lewisham Hospital

The hospital is an acute hospital with 570 beds, an 87 per cent occupancy, and out-patient attendances numbering 129 000 each year.

The HIC team concerned with the Project has remained the same except for two changes in the operational team. The original administrative member moved to a new post and was replaced in the team by his successor. Another administrative member joined when his department was being studied.

It would be fair to say that senior staff in the hospital were aware of the general problem of communication in management before the Project started. Although there have been no significant problems arising from the variety of nationalities of staff employed, the very presence of so many nurses from overseas has made the matron very concerned that they should feel able to approach her about their problems. The hospital has also had occasional disputes, seemingly over catering arrangements but, in fact, partly over communication problems.

When the Industrial Welfare Society were seeking a hospital to carry out a short survey of communications in hospitals in the autumn of 1962, our hospital, therefore, volunteered. Their short report indicated that communications were not as good as they might have been, though probably no worse than in the majority of hospitals. The result of the survey was some discussion of the problem, but no concrete proposals as to how to improve the arrangements. Such a basically obvious factor as good communication required, it was felt, simply a greater determination by senior staff to spread adequate information downwards. The relationships at the top level were good, but it was decided that the only further formal effort needed to improve communication was a hospital magazine. This started in 1963 and, except for the matron's meeting with ward sisters, remained the chief means of communicating with staff generally, although it was not edited by the administrative staff, but by staff in the group laboratory. They produced a lively magazine, free from too much 'chief officer slant', but starting as a quarterly, it gradually became more intermittent.

Joining the Project

The results of the IWS investigation, coupled with the general awareness of the need to improve the standard of hospital management, meant that the first letter about the HIC Project aroused considerable interest. It offered not merely in-

* Attended three-day appreciation course, 1965.
** Attended one-month course, 1976.
† Attended two-day appreciation course, 1967.
‡ Deceased.

vestigation of management problems in communication, but a 'do-it-yourself' exercise to put matters right.

At that time, as indeed throughout the Project to the present time, the problem had not been to recognize the need for good communication, but to judge whether the time and energy spent in 'improving' communication by means of more discussions, newsletters, conferences, and so on, is repaid by increased efficiency or, alternatively, to judge whether the same time and energy spent in another way would improve efficiency more. All the senior staff who attended the opening meetings in the autumn of 1964 were impressed by Professor Revans' exposition of the problem, but all felt the need for 'concrete' techniques for overcoming the difficulties outlined.

By spring 1965, having attended a series of meetings, we were sufficiently impressed with the statistical evidence and obvious belief in the project to agree to send staff on an appreciation course, and on a month's course to learn techniques to deal with this problem of communication. A major difficulty, however, arose over the medical representation. We had foreseen this problem and, partly as a result of participating hospitals' comments on the position, the training course had been reduced from three months to one month. Nevertheless, the problem remained that no staff other than consultants were sufficiently permanent to give the necessary continuity to the project, and no consultants felt able to devote time to a month's course or to the investigations which were to follow, particularly as the latter had been estimated to take up two days each week.

The courses

The three-day appreciation course was a disappointment. It was attended by the supporting-team members. All went with the hope of gaining greater insight into the techniques likely to be used. Instead, they felt that they received simply further expositions of the problems without getting to grips with the possible means of their solution. It was now considered, even more strongly than before, that the key to success lay in the techniques to be taught on the month's course in September 1965.

The administrative and nursing members were chosen for the month's course and, although the nurse fell ill and her place was taken by another, this mattered less than the continuing failure to find a medical member. The chairman of the group medical advisory committee had agreed to attend for two days a week if none of his colleagues were willing to go, and indeed did so during the first week. Then, a senior surgeon, who hitherto had not been approached concerning the Project because of his known pressure of work, expressed an interest. After being given the background, he volunteered to attend as much as he could of the remaining two and a half weeks of the course. His subsequent attendance meant that a senior clinician was closely involved with the detail of the Project, although his very involvement in clinical work was to make it increasingly difficult for him to devote time to the Project in the following two years.

The techniques learnt were chiefly concerned with interviewing, conduct of discussion groups, the compilation of questionnaires and the evaluation both of the results of questionnaires and of statistics generally. There was considerable discussion of problems of human behaviour in the work situation and particularly of what constituted 'morale' in a hospital. Throughout ran the thread of the need for good communication up, down, and sideways, so that staff receive the information to enable them to do their jobs effectively and to feel secure in them. Those who attended returned feeling that they had some insight into the techniques of the social scientist, but not that they themselves were capable of doing more than conducting interviews and discussions.

The attitude survey

A week after the month's course finished, the three supporting members met the three operational members to decide on the future course of action.

The operational members felt strongly that any attempt to localize communication problems would mean that the senior staff would simply be acting from their own previous knowledge of the situation in the hospital, which might be completely wrong. It was suggested that a survey of the whole hospital by means of questionnaires to, and group discussions with, a representative sample of staff was necessary to identify the communication problems.

In discussion, this suggestion quickly evolved into interviews with staff to obtain their views, not merely on communication problems, but on general problems in the hospital, in order to make an assessment of morale which could then be compared with morale in three years' time by means of a similar survey. Such interviews would need to be carried out by outside interviewers, and the advice of the central team was sought.

Further discussion with the central team led us to decide that free individual interviews were needed so that staff could speak their mind without any guidance from the interviewer. This, in turn, meant not only outside help such as that which could be obtained from another hospital, but expert help from social science interviewers. This was quickly forthcoming and, in December 1965, three interviewers spent three weeks conducting free interviews with nearly 150 staff of all grades.

Subsequent discussion of the methods used revealed three significant errors. First, the sample chosen, although for the most part at random, contained more senior staff than it should, as the lists were produced at a time when we were discussing the possibility of the interview work being cut down by having individual interviews only for heads of departments and above. In point of fact, the sample was large enough for the weighting of senior staff not to be particularly important. Secondly, the method of collecting the information in long-hand from free interviews meant that the chances of being able to carry out a repeat survey after three years were small.

The third problem also concerned the method of collecting data and was of much greater significance. In order to preserve anonymity, the long-hand notes of the interviewers could only be placed in the categories agreed between central and local teams by the interviewers themselves. This, coupled with problems of reclassification and typing the vast volume of information, meant that the survey results were not available until mid-summer 1966.

This delay in obtaining results meant that the project went cold for nearly six months and the interest of the staff began to wane. Nor, when the team saw the results, were they particularly impressed. No dramatic new areas for investigation arose and the most significant points seemed to be that:

(a) Human relationships and communication were the areas which gave most ground for criticism throughout the hospital.
(b) Most criticism about the service departments concerned the medical records, domestic, catering, and pathology departments. There was a considerable amount of comment about nursing staff problems because nurses formed a high proportion of those interviewed, but the few junior medical staff interviewed produced an inordinate amount of comment.
(c) The system for requisitioning for minor maintenance and supplies was criticized either directly or by implication.

As the summer holidays were just about to start, the team decided to feed back to each departmental head the comments concerning that department, together with the general section on human relationships and communication which affected everyone. This distribution was done, and meetings were held with all ward sisters and heads of departments at which the supporting-team members asked them to study the documents carefully, to discuss them with their staff in as objective a way as possible, and to take such action as they considered necessary to correct any faults implied by the criticisms. It was explained that after a few weeks, a project-team member would follow up to discuss matters with them but if, in the meantime, they required any further help, the project-team members would gladly give it.

Nursing staff

The supporting-nurse member of the team followed up the initial introduction of the document by meetings with sisters to discuss the comments, and then started a series of meetings with other nursing staff—something which had never been done before. Her comments give an indication of the way these meetings went.

'When I talked this over with the sisters, they were extremely good, they realized that some of the criticisms made were justified and were due to perhaps their being very busy or not spending that little time with the student nurses that they might have done. They felt that there were a number of ways in which they could help to make the staff feel happier about these things. But they also felt that some of the things the student nurses and the staff nurses had said were not justified, and perhaps they did not quite understand. But one of the chief things that was brought up by the nursing staff was that the matron had meetings with the sisters every month, but had no meetings with the rest of the nursing staff; and I must confess that this was perfectly true, It was something that I had decided many, many times I ought to, but I hadn't done, and I felt very guilty indeed when I read that the nurses realized as well as I did that this was something that should take place.

Now, I discussed this with the sisters and said, "You know, it is very difficult getting all the nursing staff together to talk to me and discuss things *en masse*. So if I can arrange to have two meetings on two days running, will you release half your staff one day and half the next day, so that everybody gets an opportunity of coming?" We decided that this could be done, and, about a fortnight after my meeting with the sisters, I asked all the nursing staff to attend these meetings.

I was amazed at the number, even the night nurses (I had it at 9 o'clock in the morning so that the night nurses could come), a very large attendance. I talked to them of the attitude survey, and I went through it with them. I tried, as best I could, to explain the reasons for these criticisms. I agreed that sometimes I was a little impatient with the sick staff, but I explained why. I said, "Very often, you know, there are a number of nurses who have a day off sick every week, and perhaps they are out on Wednesday, they come in on Thursday, and say, 'Sorry I was out yesterday, but I was ill all day', when somebody else has seen them shopping in the supermarket."

Everyone agreed that I had never been impatient with someone who was ill in the nurses' sick bay. They have also said they didn't like being moved from one ward to another, and I pointed out again the reason why they were moved: if two nurses went sick in one ward, there is still the same number of patients to be looked after, and somebody has to look after them. I felt at the end of that meeting, that perhaps, I got a little way with them.

Another thing brought up was social life. "Why can't we have more social life?" I said, "You can have more social life, you can have just as much social life as you like, but you must do something about it." I explained, "Not very long ago, only a year or two, I arranged for a dramatic society to give plays in the hospital and on the day the party arrived to give their play, there were about three people in the recreation room, and I and my staff were running round the nurses' home begging people to come, so it was decided that it wasn't wanted, but if you want it, you can have it. I will help you in any way I can, but you must do something about it yourselves." And I have found since then that they have done more about it. I have had more nurses coming to say, "I have a 21st birthday next week, may I have a party?" And we have supplied refreshments, or they have come and asked for equipment. They put on a play at Christmas time which they haven't done for a number of years, and I do feel that, in a sense, it is doing quite a lot of good to do things for themselves.

Then, I have tried to keep up the meetings with the nursing staff. I think this is very important indeed. I have met them every other month since the survey. About a year afterwards, I talked at both meetings, for quite a long time and then asked, "Do you really think that these meetings that you asked for are worth while?" And there was silence just for a second or two and I felt very despondent and thought "No", and then one nurse said, "Well, I think they're very worthwhile." Then there was a murmur of assent among the rest of them, and I said, "I don't want these meetings to be a lecture and I don't want to come here and just talk to you while you sit here and listen. This meeting has got to be a two-way traffic. When I come I want to discuss things with you, to criticize, but to suggest as well. It is not going to help any of you at all for me to just come and talk to you. I can come along to the classroom and do that, but I want us all to discuss things and to hear your suggestions." And immediately there were quite a number, some of them minor and some very worthwhile points. We have opened a new operating theatre and one of the nurses said to me, "Do you know there is no bell in the recovery room to summon the anaesthetist?" I didn't know, and I was very pleased to know and to be able to do something about it, and said so. Later, I made a point of telling the nurse who put the suggestion forward that it was now done.'

Medical records

One department which came in for much criticism from the nurses was the medical records department, a very busy and devoted group of staff who suffered from overwork and sickness, and who were characterized by high turnover.

They had their criticisms too; they mentioned the problems created by medical staff who cancelled clinics at short notice or altered timing of appointments, thereby causing 600 letters to be sent out altering appointments, or those consultants who took case notes away—and then complained bitterly because the 'records staff has lost them'. These points were made in a discussion with the supporting-medical member of the HIC team, who took them to a full meeting of the medical staff committee.

Feedback from the records department in autumn 1967 indicated that matters were much improved. Nevertheless, since the meetings with the records staff a year before, the team mounted, with the help of the central team, studies into admission and discharge procedures, messenger services, and the problems of missing case notes. These statistical assessments of the current situation produced a number of surprises, not least the fact that admission procedures were generally satisfactory, whereas the timing of discharges and the delays in sending out notes to the patients' general practitioners were often unsatisfactory. These matters were followed up with the staff concerned, to produce a system which, it is hoped, will be generally more satisfactory.

It also became clear that the money spent on agency staff, to relieve staff shortage in the department, would be better spent on employing junior clerical trainees who could be trained in all aspects of the department's work. This was done.

Requisitioning procedures

During 1967, requisitioning both for supplies and maintenance was completely reorganized. Centralization of stores has taken place, with a determined effort to give all users a complete catalogue of what is available. The old maintenance requisitions have also been redesigned to give a better follow-up of uncompleted jobs. By the time of the ward sisters' and heads of departments' meeting in September 1967, there were 'no complaints'.

General communications

Four developments, besides matron's meetings with her nursing staff, are:

(a) Bi-monthly meetings of heads of departments and ward sisters' representatives.
(b) The intermittent magazine, *Pulse*, has been replaced by a regular monthly *Bulletin of Internal News* under the same editors.
(c) A staff suggestions scheme.
(d) A thriving staff club, perhaps the most significant innovation of all.

These developments certainly seem to add up to much greater flow of information through the organization and a friendlier atmosphere which, unfortunately, is impossible to evaluate. We are currently trying to further this by improving the staff's first introduction to the hospital by means of conducted tours, and a handbook, while making it clear that the most effective introduction which the newcomer gets is from his head of department.

Evaluation

For those of us closely concerned with the project, evaluation is impossible. A trained social scientist may be able to provide objective means of assessment; the team members can only reckon the time and energy it has cost against what appears to be a 'better atmosphere' in the hospital. Even this may be self-delusion.

In our own personal assessment of our experience of the HIC Project, we make the following comments:

(a) The initial decision to conduct the attitude survey was the right one, because it has formed the mainspring for further action.
(b) Delay in obtaining the results, though almost unavoidable to preserve anonymity, was nearly disastrous.
(c) The original multi-disciplinary team has become largely administrative and nursing, with the occasional willing cooperation of the medical members. The working pressures on consultant clinicians seem to make this inevitable.
(d) It is impossible to treat the Project as a special study apart from the day-to-day running of the hospital. Therefore those concerned must be chief members of the three staff groups, the matron, secretary, and chairman of the medical staff committee or his equivalent. Even so, it is extremely difficult to maintain momentum.
(e) The essential centrality of the subject in general administration has meant that involvement of other staff has been intermittent. The educational value of the Project has, therefore, largely been absorbed by the comparatively few HIC team members.

Initially, the hope that the heads of departments' meetings might be vehicles for the full discussion of management problems was not realized, in that although the heads of departments claimed that they found the meetings 'interesting' the team were disappointed at the lack of contribution from the heads of departments themselves. As an experiment the following changes were made:

   (i) A rotating chairman was appointed from the departmental heads;
   (i) The seating arrangements were made more informal; and
   (iii) Syndicate discussion groups were occasionally used.

It is pleasing to report that following these changes there has been a marked improvement in the usefulness of the meetings and in the content of problems discussed.

The London Hospital by M. J. Fairey

The London Hospital participants

T. H. Arie**	senior lecturer in social medicine
Pamela Birleson†	house governor's assistant
Margaret Cutliffe*	deputy matron (until 1966)
M. J. Fairey**	deputy house governor
S. L. Last*	consultant psychiatrist (until 1966)
J. L. C. Scarlett*	house governor
June Swan†	administrative sister
P. H. Tooley**	senior consultant psychiatrist
Beryl Webster**	assistant matron

The London Hospital is a teaching hospital which also has a district responsibility. It has the largest out-patient department in the country (430 000 clinical attendances annually) and its out-patient load is a little under two per cent of the total out-patient load of England and Wales. The hospital has 717 beds and discharges between 16 500 and 17 500 patients per annum. The bed occupancy overall averages between 91 and 93 per cent on four days out of every seven in every week of the year. The bed occupancy of the main hospital exceeds 94 per cent.

In addition to the medical school (approximately 470 students) and the dental school (approximately 220 students), the hospital has training schools not only for nurses and physiotherapists, but also for radiographers (both therapeutic and diagnostic), domestic science students, dieticians, and dental surgery assistants, and it participates in training schemes for laboratory technicians, social workers, EEG recordists, and cardiac technicians.

The hospital first became aware of the HIC Project through the King

---

* Attended three-day appreciation course, 1965.
** Attended one-month course, 1965.
† Attended two-day appreciation course, 1967.

Edward's Hospital Fund for London. It is difficult to say what members of the team expected of the Project, since its purpose was not entirely clear. It might well be, however, that this was because they were not able to attend the two briefing sessions held at the beginning of the Project. The mystery was not noticeably dispelled during the progress of the month's course at Hastings, where a similar confusion was apparent. Members of the team formulated a working hypothesis that the aim of the Project was to instil methods by which to perceive and study problems within a large organization; and that the success of this attempt would be evaluated. In the event, this hypothesis proved to be not too far from the truth.

Choice of a project

On the team's return from Hastings, one of the medical members was absent from the hospital for a further three months. The remaining three members of the operational team discussed a number of projects and the following were those most seriously considered:

(a) *Attitude survey of a complete cross-section of the hospital.* This project was considered to be impracticable because of the size and diversity of the hospital; and the *immediate* practical value to be derived from such a survey did not seem to be commensurate with the work involved.

(b) *The role of one of the major service departments of the hospital.* One of the major service departments of the hospital appeared to be suffering, both geographically and socially, some degree of isolation from the hospital. It was considered that a survey of the staff's perception of the department might demonstrate how closer integration might be effected.

(c) *Survey of senior medical students' and junior medical staff's attitudes.* Though this problem has been extensively studied elsewhere, the team considered that it might be fruitful to study in their own hospital the difference in attitudes towards authority between senior medical students and junior medical staff a year or two years after qualifying. It was considered that the survey of overall attitudes of those within this spectrum might point up factors significant in the change. If this were the case, it might well be that some of these factors could be ameliorated by administrative measures.

(d) *Medical records department.* At the time, morale within this department was causing some concern and a survey of the staff might, it was thought, suggest methods by which morale could be improved.

(e) *Attitudes of those involved with the emergency admission of patients.* The emergency admission of patients had posed a severe problem for some years and the nursing staff in particular found the continual strain trying and not in the best interests of nurse training. An operational research survey was already in progress and an attitude survey would complement its findings.

These projects were discussed by all the members of the team and with the matron. It was considered that the hospital had sufficient overt problems to make it unnecessary at this stage to look for hidden problems that might emerge in a general attitude survey.

The survey of attitudes of senior medical students and junior medical staff, while perhaps interesting sociologically and capable of suggesting meaningful improvements, was not immediately applicable to any urgent problem facing the hospital at the time.

The major service department had been a source of some apprehension for a number of years. The reduction of its isolation would, undoubtedly, have been of benefit to the organization of the hospital. A number of problems, to some degree based on personal relationships, existed however and it was felt that the time was not appropriate to bring these relationships to a crisis.

Morale in the medical records department was a source of much concern and in other circumstances this would have been the survey of choice. The department had, however, been surveyed by a team from another hospital as part of the Hastings course. It was considered inexpedient to repeat a survey within the same department so shortly after the training survey.

On the other hand, a survey covering the whole field of emergency admissions would touch on one of the major problems facing both the medical and the nursing staff. For this reason it was felt that it was this survey which should be pursued, since it would be dealing with a problem of immediate concern to a large section of the hospital. It would be complementary to an existing survey; and the problem surveyed was of considerable importance.

Organization of the Emergency Admission Project[3,4]

The final choice of a project was made known in the first instance through the team's approach to those members of the staff included in the full survey. At the same time announcements were made to the consultants, and to other members of the medical staff, telling them of this new approach to a longstanding problem. No initial efforts were needed to attract the interest of those whose working was affected by the project. Interest in the problem was already widespread and, indeed, members of the team were struck throughout by the willingness of all those approached both to discuss the problem and to pose solutions, usually of a most practical nature.

The organization of the project devolved upon the four members of the team who had attended the month's course on social research techniques. Following the choice of project, the team met to discuss the form the inquiry should take. It was decided to undertake a pilot survey, which would be organized by the nursing and administrative members of the operational team. When they, with one of the medical members, had completed the interviews for the pilot survey (early April 1966), the team met to consider the results. From these results one of the medical members devised a questionnaire to be used in the major part of the survey. After discussion among the team, this was amended slightly and the questionnaire printed. Advice on the study design was then sought from the members of the Medical Research Council's Social Medicine Research Unit, and at this point our other medical member rejoined the team.

The nursing and administrative members determined the population to be surveyed by reference to the records, drew the appropriate sample in the one instance where this was necessary, and organized the dispatch of a preliminary letter to those chosen as respondents. In the period late April to mid June 1966, 116 interviews were carried out by the four members of the team. During the latter half of this period, the administrative member discussed with the operational research department the processing of the data collected. The computer program for analysing it was devised and the program tested. The information contained in the completed questionnaire was coded for the computer and the result subsequently analysed by the administrative member. The results were then discussed with the members of the team, who unanimously nominated him to write the report. The draft report, complete save for the concluding section, was completed with assistance from a medical member by mid July.

Both the house governor and matron were kept in touch with the progress of the inquiry by the members of their staff on the operational team. An interim report, setting out the ground covered by the pilot survey, was submitted to the house governor in mid April.

One object of the survey was to seek, from those who experienced the problems associated with the emergency admission of patients, their own solutions to the problems posed. To this extent, the survey mirrored the ideas of those involved. It should, however, be remembered that the object of the study, was the description in depth of a problem, partly to solicit suggestions and partly to inform those who had the responsibility for finding a solution.

At no stage during the survey did any member of the team experience any reaction from those interviewed which could be remotely described as uncooperative. Indeed, many of those interviewed welcomed the interviewers, and expressed hopes that their efforts might result in some radical solutions to the problems described.

Action taken in the Emergency Admission Project. In describing the action taken upon the report, it is first necessary to consider the part played by the attitude survey, the details of which have just been described. The problem to which the talents of the team were applied was one that had troubled the hospital for a number of years. The survey was complementary to a study, by the operational research unit, of bed usage and of the various phenomena associated with the pressure of emergency admissions. The role of the attitude survey, therefore, was to provide further information on a problem, the existence of which was known, and of which some aspects had already been investigated.

The findings of the attitude survey were fed back to most of those who had taken part. They were presented at two study days for staff nurses (thus covering all the staff nurses) and two study days for sisters (thus covering all the ward sisters involved). A copy of the survey was given to all the senior registrars undertaking full duty and most of the junior registrars: and a summary of the report went to every member of the consultant medical staff and the board of governors. On subsequent reflection, there was a rather startling omission in this feedback process, in that house officers as a body were not offered access to the results. A number of copies were circulated, however, to individuals known privately to members of the team.

In the discussions with the nursing staff about the results of the survey, the major points of interest lay in the social and ethical problems involved in refusing patients when the hospital was full or, alternatively, of not refusing them and the subsequent necessity of putting up extra beds in the wards. Many of the sisters, in particular, appeared to be impressed by medical staff arguments for extra beds; and there was a noticeable absence of interdisciplinary recrimination. In discussing the results of the survey with medical staff, there was a similar absence of this reaction.

Overall, both in the results of the survey and in the feedback discussions, it was encouraging to observe that both medical and nursing staff were profoundly concerned with the same problem and attempted, in general, to meet the same aims—although their respective professional spheres gave them different perspectives on essentially the same process.

During the period of the feedback meetings (September to December 1966), a multi-disciplinary working party convened by the house governor, with the approval of the medical staff, had been considering what remedial measures could be taken. The members of the working party had the findings not only of the attitude survey but also of the statistical study carried out by the operational research team. A number of measures were considered and suggestions were formulated for discussion by the standing committee of the medical staff. At this point, however, events overtook this ordered process of consideration.

In the latter half of December 1966, and more particularly in the early part of January 1967, the pressures had been extremely high (on 11 January the occupancy in the hospital was 99·04 per cent). The combination of this continuing pressure and shortage of nursing staff was such that it was considered that the problem should be discussed with the chairman of the hospital. At a series of discussions between the chairman, the matron, and the house governor, it became apparent that if some control could be exercised on admissions from the waiting-list, it might be possible to alleviate the pressures arising from the high but unpredictable level of emergency admissions. The nursing and administrative members of the team were instructed to devise a system using the simple principle that the number of patients to be called for admission should not exceed the number of patients who would be discharged on any given day. This principle could be further refined in that an allowance could be made representing the average number of patients who might be admitted as emergencies on a given day.

They devised a system in which the ward sisters, in consultation with the registrars of the firms concerned, would predict the number of patients to be discharged for each one of the seven days in advance of the day on which the prediction was made. No firm could send for more patients than the number predicted as due for discharge three days ahead. On the basis of the predicted discharges three days ahead, patients on the waiting-list were warned that they

139

were coming near the time of their possible admission into hospital. As a further safeguard, patients were asked to telephone the hospital, at first on the day of their admission, but latterly on the afternoon preceding the admission, to check whether their bed was still available.

This system was introduced gradually throughout the hospital from mid February to mid July 1967. It was introduced in this piecemeal fashion to enable the two operational members to discuss the scheme and its implications individually with every member of the medical and nursing staff directly involved (a total of approximately 95 medical staff and 26 nursing staff).

Further studies

Between April and June 1968, a second attitude survey was carried out among the same section of the hospital and covering the same topics that had appeared at the first survey. In general, there were highly significant changes of attitude in all those areas where alterations to the system had been made. In marked contrast, in the one area where no changes had been carried out, there were no overall significant changes of opinion: indeed, opinion remained remarkably stable.

At the same time, the prediction system was evaluated. The capacity of ward sisters to predict discharges was high for events occuring as far as two days ahead. Thereafter, as might be supposed, this capacity decreased. The most common fault encountered was the omission of predictions relating to a particular patient. Predictions made on surgical wards were significantly better than those on medical wards. Concurrently with this work, an intensive study of many parameters affecting the operation of the hospital in the period between the two attitude surveys showed that the external pressures upon the hospital had remained very much the same. The number of cases discharged had increased and hospital occupancy had remained stable Internally, the lodging rate had decreased significantly: and the study showed that one of the major factors in this decrease had been the prediction system.

Organization of the Visiting Hours Project.[5] The second project upon which the team embarked was in no way connected with the first. In the later months of 1966, the medical and nursing staff had agreed to an alteration in the visiting hours. This particular project had been sponsored by the medical/nursing liaison committee, which subsequently asked the team to survey the effects, on both staff and patients, of the proposed alteration. The committee intended that this survey should be one of the factors on which the new visiting hours would, within a six-month period, be evaluated.

Members of both medical and nursing staff were informed that the survey would be carried out. All respondents received a letter from members of the team explaining the project and enclosing a questionnaire.

The team discussed the form the survey should take and decided that it should consist of a 'before and after' inquiry. The medical member devised a questionnaire and the other two members organized its dispatch to members of the staff.

140

The administrative member and a number of the medical students drew a sample of patients and organized the distribution of the questionnaire to them. The second part of the survey was organized in a similar way using the same questionnaire. The completed questionnaires were classified and transcribed for the computer. The medical and administrative members subsequently analysed the results and wrote the report.

It was the aim of the survey to seek the opinions of those affected by the change and the questionnaire was so constructed that comments other than those directly solicited could be made. In this way, a number of alterations were put forward by the respondents which were, of course, taken into consideration in the report.

When the report was completed, it was presented to the medical/nursing liaison committee with whom lay the responsibility for recommending, first to the medical staff and subsequently to the board of governors, what further action should be taken. The team's connection with the problem ceased at this point, though the administrative member of the team was subsequently concerned with the implementation of the policy decided by the board of governors, on the recommendation of the medical staff.

Conclusions

In the view of the team, the HIC Project in the hospital has proved successful. A number of specific gains have been made and lessons learned. A major overall gain has been in experience of a multi-disciplinary approach to problem-solving. This approach had already been employed at the hospital in a major study of the reduction of errors in the administration of drugs, a project which started in approximately September 1965. The experience gained by the team has strengthened the view that this approach is of value in the solution of hospital problems, and has widely extended the use to which this method might be applied.

The experience gained in the emergency admission study has demonstrated conclusively the value of a study in depth of a particular problem for those who are responsible for seeking solutions to it. The Project has alerted the interest not only of the team, but also of the upper levels of management, in the value of quantitative analysis of major aspects of hospital functioning. It should, perhaps, be noted that such analysis is facilitated by the existence in the hospital of a computer unit. It may well be that such analysis would prove extremely difficult if these facilities were not available.

The disparate nature of the two surveys conducted by the team has made it possible for members to consider the circumstances in which this approach to hospital problems would most profitably be used. The Emergency Admission Project carried out a specific task in the description in depth of a problem that affected the overall running of the hospital. The members of the team were responsible for the feedback of the information obtained and two members were subsequently responsible in their day-to-day duties for putting into practice a workable solution of the problems perceived during this exercise.

In the second survey, the team again carried out a specific study, the limits of which were more circumscribed than in the first survey. The team was not able to conduct a feedback of the data obtained and was not involved, except incidentally, with the implementation of the policy finally decided.

On balance, the members of the team consider that, in studies related to areas where there are specific responsibilities or already hardened opinions, it is more difficult to feed in observations and ideas than in areas where there is no specific responsibility involved or where there are no preformed attitudes. It is possible to conclude, pessimistically, from this that there is room for surveys of this sort only in non-controversial and, therefore, conceivably, unimportant matters. The team's experience, however, leads its members to believe this is not the case. Their work has been a fruitful source of collaboration between the disciplines and has shown that this collaboration is effective in an increasing number of areas within the hospital. The team is heartened by the collaboration so far received from those whom it has studied; and it is fair to observe that the techniques emphasized during the Hastings course are now regarded as normal aids to management that can be compared with other aids, such as, for example, the computer and operational research.

North Middlesex Hospital by W. Alderson

North Middlesex Hospital participants

W. Alderson**	assistant group secretary
B. Chant	group catering officer
C. A. R. Evans*	group secretary
Kay Kenrick*	matron
G. S. A. Knowles*	consultant anaesthetist
A. Smith	deputy hospital secretary
Pamela Steele**	deputy matron

My introduction to the HIC Project was gained at the one-month course I attended as the operational-administrative member of our team.

Although there had been a three-day appreciation course at which the three supporting members of each hospital had been briefed on the aims of the Project, I found difficulty in trying to assess what effects the Revans teachings might have on hospital routine and, therefore, joined the course with an open mind on the benefits that might be derived from applying them at my own hospital, a district general hospital of just over 700 beds.

On return to normal hospital duty after a month spent trying to assimilate a myriad of facts and figures on subjects most of us had heard discussed for the first time, the hospital team set a date to meet and determine where we should try out our newly acquired techniques. We soon discovered that the intervening Christmas festivities had done nothing to improve our memories, and because

* Attended three-day appreciation course, 1965.
** Attended one-month course, 1965.

142

we had but a short time to practise what we had been taught at Hastings, we decided to repeat at our own hospital the exercise that three of us had already carried out at The London Hospital as our test-piece for the course, namely a study of staff wastage in the medical records department. Although we recognized the need to brush up on survey methods, this study was not to be quite the academic exercise the reason behind this decision would suggest, for the records department had long been plagued by a very high turnover of staff, which had at one time caused the administration considerable concern.

We embarked on our survey by interviewing a one-in-ten sample of staff, using free interview methods, and from the material thus obtained formulated a questionnaire for completion by the entire records staff. The topics raised by the interviewees fell into four main categories:

(a) communication
(b) management and organization
(c) conditions of employment
(d) amenities and welfare

The questionnaire the staff were asked to complete listed 18 questions, each having a positive and negative statement, two single questions, and one calling for comment on any one specific aspect of job content upon which there was very strong feeling. Analysis of completed questionnaires revealed that the amenities and welfare aspects of the hospital were poorly regarded, whereas management and organization were, generally speaking, well thought of. Communication and conditions of employment attracted only moderate scores. Despite the fact that the records department had been the subject of a number of fact-finding studies in the past, the staff were most helpful and enthusiastic in their attitude at the questionnaire stage. Several reasonably significant factors emerged from the project and the team met to discuss the categories of action into which these fell and how best to tackle them.

As we saw the problem, some of the minor questions were capable of solution through administrative action, but there were others that lent themselves to further involvement of the records staff, and, as a first step to staff participation in the project, we called a meeting of the entire records personnel so that we could feed back the information they themselves had given. Only 50 per cent of the departmental staff attended and, although they listened with interest to the findings of the survey team, they showed no desire to become involved with the problems it had highlighted, and attempts to get a small sub-group going among them met with little response. Generally speaking, they took the view that none of the matters mentioned was new to them and it was not necessary for them to take part in discussions on how remedial action should be applied.

However, we were able to get a small three-person team set up to look into the re-siting of an inquiry desk installed in the entrance hall of the out-patients department. The staff had said the desk was badly located, thus causing undue pressure on another section of the department which had to answer many inquiries that should not have been addressed to them. But even this small measure of self-help was given reluctantly and further attempts to involve staff in the project were unsuccessful. What steps could be taken to remedy the problems of the records department had to be taken by straightforward administrative action.

The medical records survey, however, brought to our attention the poor regard the staff had for the hospital's amenities, and we felt that this was an area we should look at in more depth.

Because of the rapid growth of the departments employing professional and technical staff, we had been faced with a number of problems associated with their messing and other welfare arrangements, and we thought it would be worthwhile to sound out their opinion on the hospital's amenities and welfare. We realized that this could well develop into a fairly extensive study and a call for a pilot survey before putting a questionnaire to the entire staff; this we knew we could not undertake unaided. The central team were asked for help and they agreed to get the study under way with the aid of some students to do the spadework. Unfortunately, although preliminary arrangements had already been made for group interviews, illness and other commitments badly depleted the central team, compelling us to confine what was to have been a full-scale study to very limited individual interviews with twelve of the professional and technical staff. Even so, this exercise kept one member of the central team fairly busy for a week or two. The scored summary of interviews was used as the basis for the feedback discussions which we subsequently held with the staff. From the answers given to the six set questions put to them, the consensus of opinion which emerged from the feedback meetings was that these members of the professional and technical staff felt something should be done to improve communications and catering arrangements.

It was felt that the present methods of disseminating information were inadequate now that the hospital group had become so large (the merging of two former groups had produced a group of ten hospitals with some 2400 general beds). This resulted in the presentation of *faits accomplis* rather than the passing on of matters for consideration. It was therefore decided that regular senior staff meetings should be held, at which the administration would make known as many as possible of the forward planning proposals for the hospitals, thus giving opportunity for prior consideration of these as far as practicable. On the question of catering arrangements, it was agreed that the present pattern of use of facilities available was so confusing that nothing short of an extensive review of these arrangements would serve any useful purpose.

We saw this as a project on far too big a scale for the hospital team to tackle alone and again decided to seek the help of the central team. And, as usual, the answer to our request for help was an immediate and enthusiastic Yes. At this stage the central team were anxious to establish connections for the hospital teams with universities and colleges and it was felt that this was a propitious moment to set up such a liaison with the local college of technology. One or two members of both the central and hospital teams met at the college with a view to involving them in the proposed catering project. We were all most heartened by the promises of help we received from the college staff and went back to the hospital to outline to our colleagues the first steps we had agreed with the college to get our study under way. The central team made available a student and he arranged to live at the hospital and to eat in each of the five messes, dining-halls and canteens to get staff views on general catering matters. A number of weeks were spent gathering this information and details of the current pattern of messing, and then we felt able to make a start by formally interviewing a random sample of staff. These interviews were of a group nature with staff of the following categories:

medical staff
sisters and charge nurses
student and staff nurses
nursing auxiliaries
professional, technical and clerical staff
ancillary staff

Each of the groups nominated a reporting officer from among themselves and each was led by a member of the central team or of the college staff. Reports of these meetings were studied by all three teams with a view to getting from them matters upon which to base a questionnaire. But although the criticisms made about the catering service were interesting, they did little to point to the type of service staff would like to see provided. However, immediate action was taken to resolve some of the difficulties encountered by staff in the dining-halls, and since many of these involved faulty or insufficient supervision, steps were taken to reorganize supervising arrangements so that complaints could be dealt with more speedily and effectively. But we were still no nearer to bringing about rationalization of messing, or finding out what the hospital staff really wanted, and it was this sort of information we required if we were to undertake a complete reorganization of our catering facilities. To bring this about, we set up a small steering committee whose job it was to draft a questionnaire for the full HIC team's approval.

The approved questionnaire covered, broadly speaking, value for money and quality of service and food, and sought information on whether staff were prepared to eat in a mess hall used by all grades of staff wherein could be obtained a wide range of meals which could be purchased as separate constituent parts. Before submitting the questionnaire to the entire staff, we decided to put it to the six groups of interviewees for their comments on its content and wording so that we could revise them where necessary. A few amendments were made as a result of this pilot run, and we then sent the questionnaire off to all 1360 members of the staff for completion.

While awaiting the return of completed questionnaires, members of the central and hospital teams and the college staff met to discuss the scope of the analysis and to make arrangements for the measuring of our eating-places so that we would have an idea of their capacity and how they could be used to meet the wishes of the staff as reflected in the completed questionnaires.

A total of 648 questionnaires were returned by staff, a response of 47 per cent. The analysis of our survey was produced by the computer at Enfield College of Technology, and the combined team held several detailed discussions to determine a line of possible action arising from the information provided. But because voting on questions relating to patterns of messing and revised requirements was fairly marginal, it was decided to draw on a Management Research Study Report for guidance on how best to use our canteen/dining-hall facilities. The analysis did, however, produce some very valuable information on a number of catering and allied needs, and it is hoped to be able to follow up some of these at a later date when facilities permit.

In the meantime, the team made recommendations to relieve some of the problems highlighted by the study, although a number of the proposals made had to be amended by the senior officers to suit local requirements.

Questionnaires concerning choice of service were sent out to all staff using two of the small dining-rooms in which it was hoped to make certain rearrangements, and the indications were that a pattern of messing similar to that existing would emerge if a choice of either cafeteria or waitress service were offered. These results confirmed our views that the two small messes were capable of wider use and we therefore set about making certain rearrangements which, summarized, amounted to the provision of a second doctors' mess giving a waitress service and providing set meals, with the existing mess being adapted to provide cafeteria service and the opportunity of having separate parts of meals against cash payment.

It is hoped that these measures will overcome the long periods of waiting the medical staff has had to face at lunch-times and enable us to cater for the fairly large increase in medical staff that will accompany our new major building project. Reducing the numbers to be fed in the cafeteria mess will also mean that for the first time we shall be able to provide after-lunch lounge facilities, for which the junior staff have been pressing for a number of years.

The senior staff dispossessed of the small mess, which is now to become a waitress-service mess for medical staff, are to be accommodated elsewhere and will retain the choice of eating by waitress or cafeteria arrangements.

We hope that a further outcome of the study will be the ability to extend messing facilities to a number of other senior staff for whom they were not formerly provided, and steps are being taken to cater for these people in the waitress mess and, possibly, also in the central cafeteria mess by planned staggering of meal-times.

The details of the survey and its financial implications were considered by the management committee to whom a plea was made, on behalf of the combined team, that it make every effort to obtain much larger central catering/rest-room facilities in order that these may be used by the entire staff.

These rearrangements took effect from 1 March 1969, and we look forward to a considerable improvement in the service when things get under way.

So far, however, the sum total results achieved from our efforts are not very impressive. Indeed, the team would be the first to admit that they have done less than they would have liked. This is not, however, due to lack of willingness, for I think we are probably as anxious as any to make full use of the techniques acquired at Hastings in 1965. But although at that time we were convinced that we could devote a fair proportion of our duty and free time to the carrying out of HIC Projects, this did not work out in practice. The varying duty hours worked by the multi-disciplined team in themselves posed a number of problems and made it most difficult to assemble many members at any one time. We have to admit that the team met neither frequently nor regularly, but we realize that this problem is not peculiar to our hospital. It is doubtless exacerbated by the fact that our team is made up of the most senior members of each discipline which, of necessity, limits the chances of getting them all together. Attempts have been made to overcome this by involving junior staff in project activities but, except in the case of the catering survey, all efforts in this direction failed. It is possible that we have been a little more successful in obtaining staff participation in the catering survey for, whereas our previous studies were among only limited categories of staff, the catering project affected every person employed in the hospital, and thus widened our scope.

Perhaps the outstanding feature of both our earlier studies was the general lack of enthusiasm on the part of the staff concerned, combined with a certain amount of scepticism and even suspicion. It seems inevitable that honest attempts at evaluation will sometimes be interpreted as implied criticism. This is probably due to the somewhat clumsy approach by the team, but it seems that any similar survey carries with it (as far as staff are concerned) the hint that all is not well with the department under review. Perhaps what we need to achieve greater staff participation is the completion of a survey showing tangible proof of success, for it is on results that are of obvious and lasting benefit that the majority of staff judge our efforts in this field. But, alas, lack of funds has often prevented us from achieving such results and this lack, on occasions, caused the team embarrassment. It is relatively easy to highlight problems but, even when the remedy suggested is obvious from the facts gathered scientifically, financial constraints usually necessitate the administering of a palliative rather than a cure. When this approach to the problem is necessary, any interest that staff may have had in a survey disappears.

But although we can perhaps make no claim to the achievement of strictly measurable success, carrying out surveys has brought an increase in the level of staff consultation on matters affecting several departments and we see this as bringing about improved management–staff relations. And, apart from the individual studies, contact among the senior staff has been increased through the holding of regular meetings, the need for which was revealed by the small surveys held with professional and technical staff.

So although our use of HIC methods has not been very extensive, we are not entirely disenchanted, but would prefer not to undertake more than we can cope with, even though the help of experts is at our disposal. As to the future, we have hopes of being able to continue to do something to meet staff wishes in the catering field, and there are plans for a small departmental project upon which our thoughts have not yet fully crystallized.

Beyond this, we shall continue along the path already mapped out, but perhaps with diminished enthusiasm and no longer any great belief in the theory that a problem has only to be evaluated to be solved.

Additional comments by G. S. A. Knowles

It is with some difficulty that I attempt to give an account of my own participation in the HIC Project. Ideally, one would like to be as objective as possible, but inevitably one's subjective reactions creep in to affect one's judgement. Predominantly, I suppose, I share the feeling common to most people, of not wanting to admit that I have backed a loser, yet still feeling, deep down, that the Project really does have some value. In other words, I cannot escape a sense of guilt that I ought to have done better, especially when there are many people testifying to the apparent success of the scheme.

I must admit that I joined the Project with considerable scepticism. The stream of verbiage emanating from the central team overwhelmed me both quantitatively, and qualitatively, it did not matter how often I read it, I still did not understand it properly; the individual words had meaning, but when strung together, they communicated little. It was only when I listened to Professor Revans that I was fired with enthusiasm to find out what it was all about and to try to capture some of the practical benefits that would follow. Here I must state quite clearly that I have still not been able to correlate the results of the Project to date with the practical results we were virtually promised in those early days. To listen to the enthusiasts giving their introductory addresses, many of us felt that most, if not all, our problems were within sight of solution. No one can deny that staffing was one of the topics constantly mentioned, and it was actually said, no doubt with tongue in cheek, that it was possible that we had more nurses (for example) than we really needed, but that our apparent shortage was due to our not making the proper use of those we had.

My medical colleagues were sceptical right from the beginning, but I persisted in my enthusiasm and tried to help to put into practice some of the techniques learned by the team members on the Hastings long course. We very quickly came up against two snags. The first was the lukewarm reception given to our efforts by the staff concerned, coupled with their disbelief that they were being asked to participate actively in an investigation that might conceivably better their working conditions. In passing, I might add that it was very obvious to me that, while the team was prepared to give unlimited time to the project outside 'normal working hours', the hospital staff was not. The second snag was a financial one. Every approach to staff has been prefaced by remarks about shortage of money and our inability to promise any changes that involved expenditure. Each investigation or inquiry becomes merely an academic exercise under such conditions. Our one and only positive but paltry result was the moving of one small inquiry desk at the suggestion of the medical records clerks. This has now been put back to its original and presumably wrong position because the second site was a cold one, and no money could be found to remedy this!

After two years of the Project, attending meetings when I could, I suppose it is fair to say that I am disillusioned. I no longer expect dramatic results; the written reports pile up, however, and I sometimes wonder whether they are not becoming an end in themselves; and, on the whole, they are only marginally more meaningful than the original ones. My small experience with questionnaires leads me to think that these have to be worded in the simplest possible way to be understood, and that for some grades of staff, even this is too complicated. In any case, questionnaires seem to be greeted with suspicion by *all* grades of staff and often one feels that the victim is giving the answers he thinks he ought to give, rather than his true views.

To sum up: as far as I am concerned, there have been few positive results to get excited about so far. Staff of all grades tend to be uninterested or suspicious. Unless there is some money available to make the necessary changes that are suggested by an investigation, further effort is a waste of time.

References

1. Revans, R. W. (ed.), *Hospitals: Communications, Choice and Change. The Hospital Internal Communications Project seen from within*, Tavistock Publications, London, 1972.
2. See also Perkins, M. E., and E. G. Rocker, 'Nursing administration—changing patterns', *Nursing Times*, **63,** 890–894, 1967.
3. For a short account of this project see Webster B, 'Problems of the admission of patients', *Nursing Times*, **63,** 885–886, 1967.
4. A detailed report of this project is given in Fairey, M., B. Barber, and B. Webster, 'Admission procedures in a London teaching hospital', *British Journal of Hospital Medicine*, **4,** 800–820, 1970.
5. Also see Arie, T., and M. J. Fairey, 'Free afternoon visiting in a London hospital', *British Journal of Hospital Medicine*, 2, **4,** 1967.

12. Further action learning projects in the health services

In the same way that some of the ten hospitals found the study of one problem leading to another waiting to be examined, so it was for the King's Fund Centre. The method of encouraging others to learn from their own actions has now become a way of working which can meet most requests for help. And from the HIC study, one unforgettable lesson has been learned: only where people themselves feel a need can they be encouraged to question and to learn.

Coordination of services for the mentally handicapped

In 1967 staff from hospitals for the mentally handicapped were meeting to compare methods of improving the quality of life for their patients. They recognized that one of the barriers was the generally poor communication between hospital and community health services, although these two branches had responsibilities for the same patients. After a meeting in 1968 for representatives of many organizations claiming to care for the mentally handicapped, a small working party of volunteers, mainly medical officers of health, was formed. With the aid of Revans and after meeting several times during the year the working party identified the need for better communication and suggested a study to find ways of meeting it. In June 1969 the King's Fund decided to sponsor the project for at least one year, and a research officer, Ali Baquer, was appointed. The project was called *Coordination of Services for the Mentally Handicapped* and ran until December 1972. The working party, though maintaining an interest, ceased to have an official function once the research officer was appointed.

Unlike the HIC Project, this had no steering committee and no central team. One or two people were employed by the research officer on a part-time basis, when he saw the need. Seven widely scattered and varying local authority areas were invited by Revans to take part in this project. They were asked to send to a first meeting two members of local health service staff. Two hospital staff working in the same area were also invited through the regional hospital boards. Those who attended the meeting became the Research Advisory Group, taking all decisions as to the conduct of the project right up to the presentation of the final report to the sponsors. The group consisted of medical officers of health, health visitors, social workers, hospital consultants, administrators and nurses as well as general practitioners. The one general practitioner present at this first meeting, Dr Michael Spark of Gateshead, was voted chairman of the national group. The number and mixture of professionals represented at successive meetings of this group varied considerably according to location and main topic for discussion. An interesting reminder of the barrier between hospital and community was that for a time a separate hospital advisory group was maintained. When this group realized that they had cut themselves off from the main group they wondered how it had happened and how they could get back. Before they could move, however, the hospital study was curtailed through lack of funds and efforts were concentrated on finding evidence to demonstrate and action to improve the realities of communication within the seven local areas. Details of the research design and findings of this study are in the first report *I Thought They were Supposed to be Doing That*,[1] and in the two subsequent publications, *Coordination of Services for the Mentally Handicapped*,[2] and *But Surely That is their Job?*.[3] The object of this brief reference is to demonstrate progress in the involvement of people in making their own studies of their own problems: *action learning*, following from the HIC study.

The families for whom the services were provided were at the centre of the study. The aim was for the field staff themselves to discover any gaps in the local coordination of services in the seven areas, to compare results among themselves and to plan together for improvement. The varied professional staff providing the services were in control of the study, obtaining by their own efforts the facts they themselves had agreed were needed. The research officer was not 'doing the research', but remained in the background, coordinating the efforts of the seven areas and helping those in the service to find out what they needed to know, in ways which would make their evidence valid. Improvements seen as advantageous to the families in the study were implemented at once without waiting for the research programme to be completed. Each of the seven areas made use of local findings and made specific changes relevant to their area and their way of serving it. In some areas doctors, social workers and health visitors became very involved, not only with the study, but in working together. They became friends and visited each others' houses to work out strategy in a way they later declared would have been impossible before the study was started. Staff from one area visited another to demonstrate the technical ground work necessary for launching the study. Participants made the effort to keep other areas in the country informed about the study through conferences, articles and in the professional journals. Once the study was over they helped in circulating findings and talking about the study in training courses for social workers and health visitors.

It would be a mistake to think easy progress in action learning was visible in every aspect of this study. Not all those who joined the research advisory group were there from choice; some were just sent by their chief officers, and in consequence, through lack of interest or understanding, and not seldom both, contributed little. They became a hindrance rather than a help. There was a hard core of health service staff from about five of the seven areas who attended most meetings, influenced the design of the study as a whole and the progress made within their own area. Except in one or two cases, the interest taken in the study by those in command at the local authorities and the hospitals was very limited. As in the HIC Project it was as though top people were prepared to let the study be undertaken in their institution, as long as they did not have, themselves, to be involved; indeed, the suggestion that an organization should be examined in order to be improved struck some senior staff as very strange.

The implementation of the Seebohm Report[4] was started while this coordination study was in midstream. Although this did not invalidate the research findings, it did seriously impede the communication between health and social service staff. Several interested social workers withdrew from the study, claiming all their time and attention was needed to secure their own posts and implement the statutory changes. Added to these adverse factors, the initiators of the project were unable to obtain sufficient funds to continue it as originally planned. Time to analyse the findings therefore was very short and so this task was regretfully not shared with the health service staff in the areas. The majority of them had to be content to accept the findings as presented, recommend action at local level and decide what of the information collected should be included in the final report. Nevertheless, the study demonstrated what it was hoped the HIC Project would also have done: not only that organizations can engage their multi-disciplinary staff in examining their own actions, both individual and collective, and the consequences of them, but also, that given expert research resources and good coordination (rather than control), they can work together designing and accomplishing an effective common attack upon their problems.

Nurses' attitudes to patients

Running parallel with the above study in coordination, but concentrated at the King's Fund Centre, was an attempt to encourage nurses to study their own attitudes towards their patients. It was hoped that, by thinking more about how and why they behaved, the nurses might gain a greater insight into their own work. Two groups of approximately 80 nurses from non-teaching general and psychiatric hospitals had the opportunity to attend meetings at the King's Fund Centre one day a month for six months. Reports of these meetings were widely circulated.[5] Dr Tom Caine, consultant psychiatrist at Claybury Hospital, was able to demonstrate some shift towards a more liberal attitude in the nurses as a result of their attendance at these meetings, but there was no evidence of a similar change in attitudes among staff in the same hospitals who did not join the exercises. Senior nurses invited to evaluate the effect of the first year's six study days asked the Fund to continue along similar lines with their neighbouring hospitals. They wanted local discussions, in the belief that nurses from other hospitals needed the same initiation. The senior nurses asked also that in future nurse administrators and tutors be invited to join the bedside nurses in their discussions. In the second year's study an attempt was made to meet these requests of the senior nurses. During the third year a fresh effort was made to encourage the hospitals themselves, rather than the King's Fund, to sponsor the study.[6]

Having given virtually all the London hospitals the opportunity of joining in the previous study, the King's Fund then chose seven widely differing hospitals on the outskirts of London, and, instead of two nurses being detailed to spend a day at the King's Fund Centre for discussion on attitudes, six nurses were chosen to form a team within each hospital. It was their task to study, in a manner of their own choosing, attitudes to patients in their own hospitals. They attended together at the King's Fund Centre once a month to compare notes with teams of bedside nurses from the other six hospitals undertaking the same task. These teams were each supported by two senior nurses in the same hospital. A special effort was made to transfer the responsibility for the study from the King's Fund to these senior nurses. They were all locally visited and, having agreed to participate, were invited to meet at the King's Fund Centre to discuss how they thought the teams could work within their own hospitals, what exchanges of information there should be between hospitals and what should be circulated within individual hospitals. This meeting was repeated towards the end of the study, when the senior nurses compared the effects produced in each hospital and approved the plans of the bedside nurses for a conference to explain their work and how they had set about it.

Some teams progressed much more satisfactorily than others. Nurses from the general and psychiatric field expressed a conviction at early meetings that they had little in common and still less to compare. But gradually, with more understanding, came the realization that they could learn from each other something about their approach to patients as people. At the end of nine months the teams presented their projects, and confirmed the value they put upon them, to an audience composed mainly of very senior nurses from all over the country. The teams spent the last of six meetings designing the programme, and incidentally electing their own chairman for the day, a student nurse from a hospital for the mentally handicapped. It was stimulating for this audience of senior people to observe how ably the young student conducted the conference and allocated, without fear or favour, the opportunity to speak.

Behind the scenes, and throughout these three years of observing nurses' attitudes, were five nurses, a psychologist and two experienced health service research workers. This team endeavoured both to ensure that learning took place and to identify what made it possible. They tried to strike a balance between 'letting things happen naturally', and making sure that as many as possible were stimulated to take part. When the separate studies of the hospitals began, in the third year, the two research workers had unfortunately moved out of easy reach of London, although the hospitals still badly needed their advice whenever the teams encountered lack of interest in, or even open hostility to, their efforts to involve others in the studies. They also wanted research techniques, not only to ensure the validity of their findings but to support their own confidence in what they were trying to achieve. Much laborious effort was expended by this residual team to interest personally the senior staffs at the hospitals whose bedside nurses were so bravely carrying through the agreed projects. And as with the coordination study among the services for the mentally handicapped, hindered by the implementation of the Seebohm Report,[4] so were the teams in this project continually frustrated by the game of blind-man's-buff set off by the Salmon Committee.[7] The entire nursing administration of the hospital system was undergoing change of a character that precipitated conflict and opposition, not only between nurse and nurse, but also between nurse and doctor. Nursing administrators, we were constantly reminded, now had to give their time to matters altogether more lofty than the provision of patient care. And so, from the original seven, two hospitals only remained loyal to their mission; in the one, the senior nurse continued with encouragement and help for her juniors; in the other, the administrator showed her professional touch by keeping actively involved with her study team at the bedside. These two hospitals sets have continued to monitor their own attitudes to patients and have now established teams of diversified workers dedicated to improve patient experience both in hospital and before or after being there. One objective of this programme at least seems to have been attained: to make the profession more generally aware of attitudes as a topic of debate and as a channel for ambition. We may lack scientific proof that these two teams have achieved all they would hope for, but they have had some reward in the attention that their studies have attracted throughout the hospitals of Britain. From the General Nursing Council, no less than from individual hospitals, medical schools, community nursing and midwifery groups, the demands to know more about this tenacious exercise in self-disclosure have become sustained, detailed and now world-wide.

It is also clear, nevertheless, from this attempt to promote a deeper awareness of nurses' attitudes that many junior nurses are still afraid of their seniors. But no less important, perhaps, is it also clear that many senior nurses now know and regret this. It is as though authoritarianism is so much the prop of hospital administration that to modify it without dismantling the machine and starting afresh seems impossible. Perhaps, now that the nurses themselves have made their diagnosis, action learning projects running simultaneously in separate hospitals for several years would be an alternative therapy. As in previous studies, this examination of attitudes has shown that it is relatively easy for managers to consent to projects in which their staff assume a place, but unless they themselves become involved, no useful outcome is likely.

The HIC Project reviewed

From 1972 to 1974 a group of administrators, doctors and nurses who had been engaged in the HIC study held a series of meetings. The object of the meetings was to examine any effect of the project upon themselves and the hospitals in which they were working at the time. How, for example, could they measure such effects? One way was to look at changes in the length of patient stay during the project in these hospitals, and to compare them with changes of patient stay in other hospitals. An account of this research is given by Drs Kenneth and Margaret Ulyatt in Part Three of this book.

There were those present at the meetings who questioned the validity of length of stay as a true measurement of improvement in hospital care. Discussions around this point led to the idea of trying to follow patients through their total hospital experience. This, it was suggested, could be done if a method of recording all patient-centred activities could be found which would identify factors affecting length of stay. As a first step, a nursing worksheet was devised in four of the hospitals whose staff comprised the majority of those attending the meetings. The nurses involved in designing and using these worksheets agreed they were a useful management tool. They were, however, unable to design a single worksheet suitable for all wards in all general hospitals, and, as some common reference is desirable for evaluating care in all hospitals, the decision was taken to interest a wider audience in the work done through these meetings, and not to proceed further with local studies for the time being.

In one of the four hospitals the doctors and nurses were interested in the length of stay of patients in their hospital as it affected the domiciliary health services. They were looking for a system of recording which would describe the care the patient received both before admission to hospital and after being discharged. This involved the hospital staff in meetings with general practitioners and community health staff, and it has already emerged that meaningfully to record the care of the patient both inside and out of hospital presents a major challenge in research design. A project entitled *General Practice, Hospital and Community* has thus been outlined. Further details are being worked out by hospital doctors and general practitioners in several different health districts. The method of conducting the project will broadly follow the study of the coordination of services for the mentally handicapped. "What total care does the patient receive and what should be done about any gaps in it?" . . . The meetings which led up to this study were, once more, significantly influenced by the reorganization of the health services in April 1974,[8] and the meetings held to design the project have been similarly confused by the unfamiliar structures in which people now find themselves working after the reorganization. Should this study eventually come into being, besides whatever may be discovered about the care of patients, we can look for more insight into action learning. How, for example, do we involve equally those at management and at shop floor levels? How do we learn against a perpetually changing background of administration? What is required to stimulate those who seem reluctant to learn or to face the discomfort of understanding themselves . . . especially those so keen on teaching others?

References

1. Revans, R. W., and A. Baquer, *I Thought They were Supposed to be Doing That, a comparative study of the coordination of services for the mentally handicapped in seven local authorities*, June 1969 to September 1972, THC 72/735, King's Fund Centre, London, 1972.
2. Revans, R. W., and A. Baquer, *Coordination of Services for the Mentally Handicapped, an account of a King's Fund research project*, by Leslie Payne, King Edward's Hospital Fund for London, 1974.

3. Baquer, A., and R. W. Revans, *But Surely That is Their Job? a study in practical cooperation through action learning*, pp. 71, ALP Publications, London, 1973.
4. Seebohm F., (Chairman), *Parliamentary Report of the Committee on Local Authority and Allied Personal Social Services*, p. 370, Cmnd. 3703, HMSO, London, 1968.
5. Boorer, David, *A Question of attitudes, an account of the first series of meetings held at the Hospital Centre from April 9 to November 11 1970; An account of the second series of meetings from October 1968 to January 1970*, pp. 30 and appendixes, THC reprint no. 519, King Edward's Hospital Fund for London, The Hospital Centre, London, 1971.
6. Boorer, David, and Shirley Hardy, *Attitudes and Assessment, an account of how teams of nurses from six hospitals came together to design projects to help them understand more fully their attitudes to their patients and to each other*, pp. 50 and appendixes, THC reprint no. 736, King Edward's Hospital Fund for London, King's Fund Centre, London, 1973.
7. Salmon, B., (Chairman), *Ministry of Health and Scottish Home and Health Department Report of the Committee on Senior Nursing Staff Structure*, pp. 205, HMSO, London, 1966.
8. Revans, R. W., *General Practice, Hospital and Community, a project proposal*, Paper II, revised August 1975, pp. 14, Altrincham.

PART THREE

An evaluation of the HIC Project
by Kenneth and Margaret Ulyatt

13. An evaluation of the HIC Project

The need to know what happened

It would have been ridiculous to embark upon such an expensive scheme as the HIC Project without any intention of making an estimate of the results. However it was not until May 1966, nine months after the project started that 'an evaluator was appointed to work independently of the Central Team to assess the effects of the Project.'[1]

The HIC Project was seen as 'an action research project, encompassing not only learning about organisations or changing things, but also acting in ways that would lead to practical concrete benefits'.[2] The evaluator hoped that 'developments would lead to internal improvements in the hospital system that would in turn help to improve the general level of functioning of each hospital'.[3]

All concerned with the Project were anxious to discover whether improvements had, in fact, occurred in the hospitals' performances. The difficulty lay in deciding what criteria and measurements could be used and how much these could be trusted to give a true estimate of performance. In the original studies in Lancashire hospitals Revans had found considerable correlation between low wastage amongst nurses and short stay, indicating rapid cure, among the patients. These two statistics were used by the independent evaluator, as well as the observation of staff absence. The evaluator was aware that the simple contrasting of variables between quarter and quarter would be extremely misleading and it is difficult not to agree with his conclusion that 'there is an important potential source of error in each of these simple comparisons'.[4] The evaluator looked particularly for long-term effects; and for differences between changes between variables occurring in corresponding quarters in two successive years. To such changes he attached considerable importance and felt that 'any demonstration of HIC effects by these complex comparisons (the change between two comparable variables at a year's interval) must be given great weight, for both seasonal and long term distortions in the data are reduced to a relatively low level'.[5] However, the evaluator (Dr Weiland) realized that he was labouring under an enormous disadvantage as he had complete statistics only up to the end of 1967, as the Project began then to draw to a close, and the books about it were commenced during 1968. Thus he had data for the previous three years of which the first was neither a full year of project work nor a control. Those hospital staffs which had been learning enthusiastically to study their organizational problems during the years of the Project might reasonably be assumed to have continued working in the same way after its conclusion. Should this be a beneficial method of dealing with difficulties, a greater lapse of time ought to demonstrate improvements more clearly, especially because changes in large institutions take some time to be seen to have occurred and to make their effects felt. For this reason an estimate of improvement in the hospital performance for some years after the end of the Project may be considered a reasonable estimate of the latter's success or failure. However, it is obvious that changes beginning prior to the Project's commencement may also be producing long-term effects, and observations from the few years immediately preceding the Project should be added to the picture in order to obtain an idea of any previous trend. It is now possible to study statistics for the years 1962 to 1971 for all the hospitals concerned.

Comparing like with like

The HIC Project involved ten hospitals in and around Greater London from 1965 to 1968. Of the participants, most were large general hospitals carrying out commoner varieties of work but three were in special categories. One of the three was a mental hospital, another a hospital for sick children and also for mentally handicapped children, and the third a large teaching hospital having district hospital responsibilities in the east end of London. It is clear that comparisons between these three and the other seven cannot legitimately be made. In the seven hospitals there are six major clinical specialties represented—General Medicine (shown in Tables 13.2 and 13.3 as GM), Paediatrics (PAED), General Surgery (GS), Trauma and Orthopaedic (T & O), Gynaecology (GYN) and Obstetrics (OBS). Length of stay in these specialties was used to assess performance not merely because the six clinical divisions were comparable between the hospitals, but also because they account between them for more than three-quarters of the clinical activity taking place in their wards and out-patient departments.

As the Project went on, two of the seven hospitals seemed to find it increasingly difficult to believe that their activities were useful and after its conclusion said as much in a public report.[6] This report, made long before the statistical analysis below, adequately demonstrates the differences between these two and the five remaining hospitals, as their teams describe their perceptions of participation in the Project. It is absolutely evident that the two 'rejecting' hospitals saw the Project differently from the 'accepting' five.

Trends towards shorter patient stay

There is, throughout the country, a general tendency to shorten hospital stay. In view of this, changes in the HIC hospitals' length of stay must be compared with some average. The regional hospital boards, which at the time of the Project were the authorities in overall charge, calculated yearly a regional average stay

160

for all the six major divisions of work in which changes can be considered in the Project hospitals. It is therefore a simple matter to compare any hospital's performance with its own regional average. Table 13.1, below, compares the average stay for the N.W. Metropolitan Region in general medicine with the performance of the medical division of hospital I, which may be regarded as a typical acceptor of the Project.

At hospital I the mean annual average of stay from 1962 to 1965 was 23·60 days. For the years 1966 to 1971 it was 20·12 days. Hence an average reduction of stay of 3·48 days occurred between the beginning and end of the Project. In N.W. Metropolitan Region as a whole the mean annual average stay for the two corresponding periods shortened by 2·13 days. Hence the performance of hospital I shows an improvement relative to the regional trend of 3·48−2·13 days, or 1·35 days on the average for each medical in-patient. Since there are annually over 3000 patients treated in the category of general medicine, it appears that after the date at which hospital I entered the Project its annual performance became better than that of its Region as a whole by about 4200 patient days.

This comparison between the change in hospital patient day stay and the appropriate regional average may be extended to all the six major categories of work listed previously, for all the seven general hospitals taking part in the Project. In Table 13·2 and 13·3 the five 'accepting' and the two 'rejecting' hospitals are indicated separately; their relative performances are entered in

Table 13.1

Mean lengths of stay (in days) of general medicine patients at hospital I, and for the NW Metropolitan region as a whole, for years 1962–1965 (before the HIC Project), and 1966–71 (during and after the Project).

Year	Hosp. I	NW Met. Region
1962	23·1	19·6
1963	21·9	19·3
1964	24·6	19·4
1965	24·8	19·1
Mean 1962–5	23·60	19·35
1966	22·6	18·5
1967	21·3	18·2
1968	20·1	17·6
1969	20·2	16·8
1970	18·6	16·2
1971	17·9	16·0
Mean 1966–71	20·12	17·22

Source: SH 3.

hundreds of days, with a minus sign for relative patient days annually saved and with a plus sign for relative patient days annually lost. The top left hand entry of −42 thus states that general medicine at hospital I shows a mean annual gain, or improvement, of 4200 days.

Table 13.2

Hundreds of patient days gained (−) or lost (+) relative to average length of stay in corresponding regions, by five 'accepting' hospitals and six clinical divisions.

Clinical Division	'Accepting hospital'				
	I	II	III	IV	V
GM	−42	−77	−55	+15	−2
PAED	+25	−40	−58	+ 5	−
GS	−38	−24	− 6	−75	+1
T & O	−38	+14	+20	+51	+5
GYN	+12	+ 9	− 9	−10	+1
OBS	−27	+17	−26	− 5	−

Source: SH 3.

(a) Hospital V had neither paediatrics nor obstetrics.
(b) The mean size of each of the five hospitals, judged upon the six divisions entered in the table was, in 1971, 12 400 patients annually.
(c) There are 28 entries in Table 13.2; their grand average is −12·75 and standard deviation 31·4. This average is the extent to which, during the HIC Project, these 28 hospital units improved annually upon the performance of their surrounding regions. The mean of −12·75 is significantly different from zero ($t = 2·15$ for 27 degrees of freedom), $P = 2$ per cent single tailed distribution.

Comparison between accepting and rejecting hospitals

We see a simple result. The accepting hospitals not only show an overall improvement *vis-à-vis* the other hospitals in their regions; they show a significant improvement; the rejecting hospitals show an equally impressive relative retrogression. The difference between the two grand means, of 3220 patient days per hospital division annually, is immensely significant; $P = 0·5$ per cent. It is possible that difficulties internal to the rejecting hospitals accounted for both the relative decline in performance *and* the inability of the staff to engage in the project. We thus seek further comparisons.

Comparable hospitals in and around London

The foregoing analysis has compared the performances of the seven hospitals in the Project among themselves with the corresponding regional averages. It is open to the objection that regional averages derive from the perforance of a great variety of hospitals. As each region contained hospitals of the most various size and functions, ranging from cottage hospitals to highly specialized units working to supply a regional need, regional averages of patient stay are not

Table 13.3

Hundreds of patient days annually gained (−) or lost (+) relative to average length of stay in corresponding regions, by two 'rejecting' hospitals and six clinical divisions.

Clinical Division	'Rejecting hospital'	
	VI	VII
GM	−15	+63
PAED	+12	+ 8
GS	+17	+56
T & O	− 7	−
GYN	+ 2	+17
OBS	+10	+51

Source: SH 3.

(a) Hospital VII had no traumatic and orthopaedic surgery.

(b) The mean size of each of these two hospitals, judged upon the six divisions entered in the table was, in 1971, 13 300 patients annually. This is not significantly different from the accepting hospitals.

(c) There are 11 entries in Table 13.3; their grand average is + 19·45 and standard deviation 25·9. This average is the extent to which, during the HIC Project, these 11 hospital units fell annually behind the performance of their surrounding regions. The mean of + 19·45 is significantly different from zero ($t = 2·49$ for 10 degrees of freedom), $P = 2$ per cent single tailed distribution.

perfectly comparable with those of any one hospital. For this reason an attempt was made to compare the results of the hospitals in the Project with those of a closely similar size and mixture of activities. Conditions of acceptance as comparable were that the hospitals were large and situated in the Greater London conurbation, that they treated at least 5000 in-patients annually and that at least three of the six clinical divisions studied in the Project hospitals were represented.

It was possible to identify 18 hospitals which fulfilled these conditions. Judging by the total number of in-patients treated annually in the six major divisions under consideration they are slightly smaller than the Project hospitals, as their average is 9000 patients annually as compared with the 12 700 average of the former.

A table similar to Tables 13·2 and 13·3 can be prepared for the 18 hospitals chosen for comparison. It has 99 entries with a mean, calculated by the same method as that for the five accepting and the two rejecting hospitals, of +4·62. This indicates that, among the 99 units in the 18 control hospitals, patients have a tendency to remain in hospital relatively a little longer than the regional average.

There is a great difference between a saving of −12·75 per hospital unit among the accepting hospitals and the loss of +4·62 of the 18 control hospitals outside the Project. It is, in fact, very highly significant ($t = 2·59$ for 125 degrees of freedom), $P = 0·5$ per cent. If the results of the two rejecting hospitals are added to those of the controls, the relative difference increases and for the 110 entries in this table the mean is $+6\cdot11$, giving a value of $t = 2\cdot83$ for 136 degrees of freedom.

These significant results indicate clearly that the five accepting hospitals differ from the 20 others in their ability to apply their skills and resources in order to have patients fit for discharge more rapidly. Since their staffs, buildings and general organizations differ widely, it is not unreasonable to suggest that this ability is related to their capacity to accept ideas of change, to work in a perceptive manner and to agree upon and implement innovations. This outlook may have caused them to become involved in the Project in the first place or may have developed as a result of their involvement. Whichever may have been the case the hospitals appear to have benefited from the experience.

Benefits of changes in length of stay

It can be estimated that the five accepting hospitals together saved 35 700 patient days yearly, in the six years from 1966 to 1971, which produces a total of over 200 000 patient days overall. This represents a very considerable saving in money, to be expressed in units of a million pounds. For each patient there has been an average saving of about $0\cdot6$ of a day, which amounts to approximately 4 per cent of their total stay. When it is considered that each hospital had only half a dozen people involved and that the Project was seen as competing with their ordinary commitments, this is a remarkable finding. It may be easy to reject the analysis as unsophisticated and to demand tests of greater rigour, but in the absence of more discriminating prime data no other tests are worth attempting. As Janet Craig remarks (see p. 155), a working party from the accepting hospitals has now launched an exercise in the collection of efficient clinical data.

Note by Professor R. W. Revans

There may well be other plausible explanations of the changes in mean length of patient stay in the five significantly greater than in the other twenty. For example, during the year immediately before the start of the HIC Project (1965), the five may have had some experience, now untraceable, that was of itself the origin of a significant improvement in performance over the next six years; this experience, as a side effect, may also have led the five to join the project. Or, alternatively, the changes at the five had little to do with the exercises of HIC itself (namely, a series of deliberate efforts to involve different departments or different grades of staff in examining and in improving their working relations), but, like the Hawthorne Effect, were merely a consequence of outside observers becoming interested in these particular hospitals. We can only repeat our original forecast, made in 1964: that hospitals which, of their own resolution, set out to clarify working relations between members of their staffs, will thereby so improve their programmes of care that average lengths of patient stay will be markedly reduced.

References

1. Weiland, G. F., and H. Leigh, *Changing Hospitals, A Report on the Hospital Internal Communications Project*, p. 27, London, 1971.
2. op. cit., p. 449.
3. op. cit., p. 377.
4. op. cit., p. 453.
5. op. cit., p. 456.
6. Revans, R. W., *Hospitals, Communication, Choice and Change*, London, 1971, *passim.*

PART FOUR

Progenitors and progenies—
before and since the HIC Project

by Professor R. W. Revans

14. Progenitors and progenies—before and since the HIC Project

Our earlier quotation from Sophocles may, it is hoped, absolve us from the charge that we are claiming credit for something new, even original. All we can expect to learn by reminding ourselves of what was said over 2000 years ago is how soon the truth is forgotten. Since men in general (and those responsible for the National Health Service in particular) are, however, justifiably cautious about innovation, we are, naturally enough, anxious to emphasize the antiquity of our thesis, and to prove for the notion of learning by doing a lineage of unimpeachable descent. The Apostle St James also gives us his support; he again is an early authority for the limitations of the classroom: 'Only be sure that you act on the message and do not merely listen; for that would be to mislead yourselves. A man who listens to the message but never acts upon it is like one who looks into a mirror at the face nature gave him. He glances at himself and goes away, and at once forgets what he looked like' (James, ch. 1, v. 22–4, New English Bible). Nevertheless, this evidence of maturity does not seem to make the idea of learning by doing any more readily understood and accepted; centres of education are, on the whole, poorly equipped for practical achievement, and often have no clear means of discriminating between taking action, on the one hand, and *talking about* taking action, on the other. Thus it was that our pioneering exercises in action learning were organized, not in any academic setting, but among men of affairs forced to *solve* urgent and demanding problems, not seeking merely to describe them.

The Nigerian Project

Perhaps the most interesting of these early campaigns—for out of it eventually sprang the consortium of London hospitals—was conducted in the jungles of Eastern Nigeria, where over ten years ago a score of managers worked together to save from bankruptcy the little mills upon which the local economy depended.[1] They had appealed to the regional management school for instruction in how more profitably to extract oil from the local palm trees, and the school had listened intelligently to their supplications, by admitting that it did not know but would help the managers themselves to discover. For a month the men of practice visited each other's sites, scattered over hundreds of square miles of bush, to try out in their common emergency an extraordinary range of hot and fanciful suggestions. What emerged from these febrile excursions were not only fresh and even unorthodox policies, such as to pay more, not less, to the girls who collected the fruit: the threat of closure under which the primitive industry had fallen was perceived by these hardbitten managers to be the very paradigm of action learning. First, the alternative to doing better was simply collective destitution; second, a hundred managers in all were involved and so could learn with and from each other by their joint attacks upon a common need; third, there were no approved answers to any suggestion, thus obliging its value to be determined by practical trial; fourth, these trials gave results of such immediate interest to so many practical men, standing to gain by success and to lose so much by failure, that each experiment was replicated a score of times and evaluated even more; fifth, in this multiplication of trials, each mill manager learned not only about mill management in general but also about his own personal methods and individual approach in particular. All this involvement led to a marriage of debate and action, of suggestion and trial, of theory and practice, of conjecture and refutation; any traditional distinction between knowing and doing, between brain and hand, was destroyed. This early work of the Institute of Management and Productivity at Enugu under Dr John Iboko suggested the model of the HIC Project launched two years later in London. The peculiar importance of this early exercise in the Nigerian jungle was, in the imagery of St James, not simply that messages became meaningful only in action: Enugu also demonstrated that men learn rapidly enough when they recognize their need to do so, or when the consequence of their not learning is clearly seen as their own destruction. And it also demonstrated that by their comradeship in adversity they were liberated from the shackles of self-deception; each helped his neighbour to identify his own shortcomings as an organic part of his own total embarrassment. The managers learned not only about the economy of the Nigerian jungle; they learned a little about Nigerian managers as well.

The Wisconsin Project

In another early experiment (conducted in Milwaukee, Wisconsin, shortly after and profiting from Enugu), the emphasis was entirely upon senior managers of independent enterprises learning with and from each other. After a couple of seminars on action learning experiences in Africa and in the London hospitals, the Americans launched a collective attempt to improve relations with their own immediate subordinates—an essay in action learning essentially personal in design. We may allow Professor Carl Larson of the Speech Communication Centre of the University of Wisconsin at Milwaukee to describe the experiment in his own words:

'... The project proper began with the selection of analysts from each of the participating companies, all of whom were top executive officers in the companies.

These analysts attended a two-day orientation program in which they acquired some basic interviewing skills and developed a research plan which would guide the collection of data in the participating companies. The general focus of the research plan concerned the discovery of "communication problems" between supervisors and subordinates.

After the development of an interview schedule, a pilot study in a non-participating Milwaukee company, and the selection of representative samples from each of the participating companies, the analysts returned to the participating companies and completed their interviews. *Each analyst interviewed employees of every company other than his own.* At the completion of the interviews, the analysts gathered for extensive analysis meetings in which they compiled the results of the interviews, identified both unique and common problems, and translated their findings into standard analysis form. At the completion of the analysis meetings, each company analyst (with the combined findings from all interviews conducted in his company) conferred with the appropriate chief executive officers to outline action programs directed toward the solution of the problems that were discovered in the interviews.

My own observations on this project were:

(a) The company analysts felt intensely and consistently that they had benefited greatly from the interviewing orientation program, from the opportunity to compare their own company operations with those of other companies, and from the information which other analysts provided them concerning problems within their companies.

(b) The problems identified were markedly similar from company to company and in most cases were sufficiently grave so as to represent extremely valuable discoveries for the participating companies.

(c) Participating companies have undertaken serious action programs to correct the problems which were discovered.

(d) The program was unique in that the companies discovered for themselves their own problems and were in a good position to evaluate realistically both the extent of the problems and their abilities to resolve these problems. In other words, there was little resistance to accepting the results of the interviews and very little difficulty in understanding the implication of these results. The staff of the Speech Communication Center have engaged in many research and consulting programs for business and professional organizations, but found that the usual resistance to suggestions originating from an academic instutution was missing in this project.

(e) We encountered no difficulty with any of the employees, nor were any problems created by the design or conduct of this project.'

Compared with those of our action studies at Enugu, the methods developed at Milwaukee became somewhat sophisticated, and later lent themselves to the quantitative measurement of opinion.[2] This meant that, as in the studies of hospital communications reported in *Standards for Morale*, the managers themselves could identify the principal obstructions to easy understanding and effective action. We learned, in the Lancashire hospitals, about the critical importance of upward communication: juniors need to feel able to seek the support of their seniors when, to the juniors, such support seems necessary. The Wisconsin study, backed by the expert technologies of a centre for speech communication, greatly enriched our views of how, in racing through their industrial problems, busy managers may actually confuse themselves and each other, making cooperation not easier but more difficult. One fatal weakness in a superior is, by insufficient disclosure of ultimate objectives, to force the subordinate to be dependent upon him, not only in emergency, when the subordinate would himself wish to be strengthened by the supporting hand, but also in everyday affairs, when insufficient delegation systematically deprives the subordinate of the power to act and thus of the chance to develop. Action learning, on that account, is one consequence of effective delegation, and delegation itself can become increasingly effective insofar as action learning is encouraged. Nor should it be forgotten that both superior and subordinate profit from these exchanges around the problems in hand.

The Belgian Consortia

Over the decade that has elapsed since *Standards for Morale* was first published, a number of different action learning consortia have been launched in Belgium. The earliest followed the lead offered in Wisconsin, except that the five participating enterprises were all very large, employing many thousands of workers on about 50 sites; the American firms were all small, averaging only one hundred employees each. The Belgian objective, moreover, was more specific: to study and improve the use of middle management. But the methodology was similar: each enterprise released part time a senior/middle manager to interview other managers—top, middle and supervisory—in all four enterprises other than his own. These interviews were, at first, unstructured, but as they progressed and as the managers charged with the search came to evaluate their findings, the interviews grew increasingly directed towards particular issues, particularly delegation. Eventually, the key issues of this managerial device were so sharply identified that they could be built into three sets of questionnaires, given, either in French or Dutch, to a total of about 1500 managers at the three levels in the five participating enterprises. The responses were treated by a computer and led, just as at Milwaukee, to constructive discussion of the blockages and contradictions, enterprise by enterprise and factory by factory, discovered (by operational managers themselves) between top management and middle, and between middle management and foremen. But a major problem was also identified, and one about which the study, as it had been designed, could do nothing: delegation of authority from one level to its subordinates was not seldom impossible since there seemed little, or at least insufficient, clear policy to form the substance of instructive or long-term delegation. Unless there is commitment to the future there can be no delegation even in the present, and one consequence of this lack in the Belgian firms was a constant complaint among subordinate managers of interruption from above on issues that should have been foreseen.

This result, that the extent to which the enterprises were guided by consistent and enduring policies was not seldom too slender to establish easy and confident relations within their hierarchies, was received with mixed feelings by the top managements to whom it was presented. Had it not been, this would have suggested that the consortium had achieved little of value. As it was, the result proved to be of critical importance, since it led several top managers in Belgium to ask themselves whether their own major policies were as clear to themselves, let alone to their subordinates, as they might be; some even questioned how their policies were formed. When, as a consequence of this first consortium, the crucial importance of intelligible policies as an influence upon managerial communication and hence on managerial morale had been discovered,[3] it was not difficult to interest the presidents and chief executives of enterprises outside the first consortium in the mechanisms of their own policy formation.

From this interest there has grown a second action learning consortium, best known as the Inter-University Programme, which entered its fourth cycle in 1974. The design draws upon the previous experiments in Nigeria, Wisconsin and the hospitals of London. A score of enterprises are invited to nominate a senior manager (called a fellow), preferably of such rank as chief engineer or economic adviser, who spends about eight months full time at work, in some enterprise other than his own, upon a strategic problem of concern to his receiving firm. During these eight months he spends one whole day every week in the company of the same three or four other fellows, discussing with them the problems and progress of each project treated by the group. Every month the five groups, one attached to a different university, come together for three days to discuss their collective problems and progress. The university staff provide continuity, advice and technical material where it is asked for; they do not lecture, except at the start of the programme, and even here their interventions are confined to explaining the structure of the programme and to helping the fellows with any necessary personal coaching. Otherwise the fellows learn from their own attacks upon the strategic problems, and from their debates with and criticisms of the other fellows. The processes of their own development (learning) and the solution of their problems (action) are inextricably mixed, so much so that we have been able to formulate a simple law, the Principle of Insufficient Mandate: 'Managers without authority over themselves have no authority over others.' If, in other words, a manager is unable to produce essential change within himself, or to acquire new ways of looking at his past experience (that is, a manager unable to learn), he is also unable to produce essential change in the system of which he is said to be in charge (that is, to help his collaborators to learn). By 'essential change' here is implied innovation, or the solution of non-routine problems demanding programmes of action impossible to lay down in advance and essentially singular to the specific situation to be changed. This principle leads at once to another: if any organization is to adapt to its changing environment (that is, if it is to learn to adjust) then the coalition of power in

173

charge of that organization must, in general, be ready to learn from its own experience rather than to follow the standard remedies of external consultants. In particular, it must be more than ready to learn from its experience of trying to bring *about that specific environmental adaptation*. There can be no simpler definition of action learning. (Evidence of action learning among freshmen in the business school of SMU, Dallas, suggests that about one-third are so impressed by the need to please their teachers that they have already become incapable of learning from their own operational endeavours. If this disability is carried into mature affairs, the consequences for economic and social development could well be serious.)

A third Belgian consortium now poses a most important question: 'Can a manager's own task, carried out normally at his own place of work, serve as a profitable exercise in action learning?' For the experiments in Nigeria, Wisconsin, and London hospitals, and in the Belgian enterprises so far described, all demand that the managers involved shall spend a great deal of time helping to treat the problems of firms or institutions other than their own. Is it, we must ask, essential that the routines of daily experience be abandoned before the men previously caught up in such routines are able to reappraise their work by varying them, or to vary their routines by reappraising their work? ... These questions are at the heart of a programme launched in 1973 at the Ecôle de Commerce of the University of Brussels, in which the mid-career manager stays in his own job, but meets, for one whole day a week over nine months, a group of others working and studying in the same way. This weekly meeting takes place at the university under the guidance of a full-time tutor and a number of professors; the purpose of the discussion is to enable the men to learn with and from each other as they report, one each week, on progress and problems in specific elements of their normal tasks. It is interesting to note that in the first year the intake was limited to ten managers, since the university staff had had no previous experience of action learning; the second course, starting in October 1974, was oversubscribed at 24 entrants immediately it was announced in May, so enthusiastic had been the accounts given by the pioneering ten to their colleagues elsewhere in Belgian management.

The Nile Project

Shortly after the end of the first Inter-University Programme in Belgium, an action learning experiment was launched in Egypt, in cooperation with the universities of Cairo and Alexandria. It has since been replicated in Benghazi, Libya, by Professor Saad Ashmawy of Al Azhar university, Cairo. The general design is similar to that in Belgium except that the fellows work in pairs, alternating week by week between their own enterprises and those of their nominated colleagues. To this extent the Nile Project[4] also anticipates the Brussels programme, since the Egyptian fellows are learning partly in their own jobs, partly while working on an unknown problem in some quite different concern. It is a further illustration of the general principles set forth in our discussion of the

Nigerian consortium—with the added advantage of calling for a severe cultural translation, from a European to an Egyptian setting. In taking the concept of learning by doing, of self-development by responsible involvement in the urgent problems of others, from the hospitals of London to the cotton fields and copper mills of Egypt, it was essential to strip from our syllabus all that did not convincingly identify, interpret, deploy and evaluate the fundamental thesis of action learning. But having done this, the response was more than gratifying: the general hospital in Cairo, with more beds than any in London, entered so deeply into the spirit of the programme that its nominated fellow (from the hospital supplies and purchasing division) studied for six months a problem in heavy industry, and a manager from heavy industry entered the hospital for the same period to exercise a reciprocal influence in return.

Coordinating services for the mentally handicapped

A further example of action learning that can be traced directly back to the HIC Project has more recently been published in a report entitled *But Surely That is their Job?*[5] This describes how about 150 persons involved in the services for the mentally handicapped—general practitioners, parents, mental welfare officers, members of voluntary organizations, health visitors, neighbours, teachers in special schools, among others—drawn from seven different areas of England, from Tyneside to the South Coast, came together to identify their unseen problems; to design, test and apply their own survey instruments in order to identify more closely what these problems were and how to tackle them; to try out proposed solutions and to evaluate their results; and generally to make the services better by helping each other understand them better. The new self-perceptions achieved by such action-oriented and mutual support are eloquently described by the social workers themselves in their own report. It is worthwhile, all the same, to mention here that all classes of social worker discovered how each believed the responsibility for coordination between services to belong elsewhere; it was invariably seen as the responsibility of some other profession to call in any third party. We may ask what is more important: the discovery of this depressing feature of a service for subjects so disadvantaged, so completely incapable of helping themselves, or that the discovery was made by those needing to coordinate their own efforts among themselves? This at least is true: that their becoming aware of it in an attempt to improve their collective task by examining together the experiences of their patients now implies that they will plan and discharge this task more effectively. For people who discover by their own efforts things about themselves do not need others, whether experts or not, to tell them the very same things in what is bound to be a comparatively incomplete and shadowy lesson. The same point is made in another context, by the research workers of the Rand/New York City Research Institute who spent many years seeking to apply action research (as action learning is sometimes called) to the massive social problems of the world's most affluent municipality.[6] It is is their considered view also that complex organizations cannot be changed merely by the injection of new plans or policies from above; the expert may logically persuade the coalition of power in charge of a social organization that such and such a policy will help it more economically to attain its goals, and the coalition of power may seek to put it into practice—by issuing instructions to its subordinates, or by appearing to consult them about lines of action already laid down in detail, or by sending them away on training courses designed and conducted by the same or other experts. But the Rand/New York City Research Institute concludes that only if the field staff of the social department are also engaged in the first studies of its problems, working from the outset with the experts, can positive results be expected. The likelihood of such results is still further increased if those for whom the social service is intended are also joined in the total study; this is independent confirmation of our own experience. (See also page 150 for a reference to this project by Janet Craig.)

The General Electric Company Programme[7]

We have concluded from our attempts to help the hospitals of London that the attitudes towards innovation of those in command are cardinal alike to the improvement of performance and to the fortification of morale. Hence it was that, when one of the most successful industrialists in Britain, Sir Arnold Weinstock, offered his corporation, the General Electric Company (GEC) as a candidate for self-diagnosis and auto-therapy, we were, for the first time in many years, entering the arena by the front door. In all our previous studies, the principal task had been to convince those in charge that their own staffs, given the encouragement to support each other, were capable of identifying, defining and treating not only the familiar host of problems long clamouring for attention, but also the armies of trouble that lie concealed beneath the horizons of the boardroom. Indeed, an unpublished study made in the hospitals' consortium shows that the correlation between attitudes of the power structure of the hospital and progress on the individual exercises launched within the hospital is so high that other factors can be neglected. And it is not only the energy that is consumed in needing to persuade senior management to think again about the nature of its total task; the danger is that a first half-hearted approval to involve subordinates in the treatment of their own problems may rapidly succumb to the threatening revelations of objective enquiry. Instructions to lay off may then frustrate the burgeoning hopes, leaving a second situation worse than the original. The significance of a direct approach from so powerful a figure as Sir Arnold Weinstock cannot therefore be exaggerated—and for several reasons.

Firstly, while nearly all the hospitals tried to excuse themselves by saying they were too busy, too much involved in doing things, to have time to examine carefully what those things might turn out to be if more were understood about them, it was our insistence upon *making action the focus of our educational endeavour* that attracted Sir Arnold's attention in the first place—and that has now secured the positive interest of scores of his senior executives. Indeed, the great variety of action learning exercises mounted by GEC has enabled us to summarize our talisman in words that are as relevant to the work of surgeons, gynaecologists and physicians as they are to those of electrical engineers or blacksmiths:

'*Action as the condition of learning*
The fundamental fact of this educational method is *action* as the essential task of the manager. All manner of experts and analysts may advise, forecast, recommend and so forth, but it is the manager's characteristic responsibility that, having talked to his advisers and perhaps debated their advice, he must get on and do something. To help him carry this singular load as effectively as possible is one mission of action learning; a second must enable him to learn from the very carrying of it. Educational programmes that fall short of doubly exercising the manager in his critical role fail to discriminate between, on the one hand, taking action, and, on the other, *talking about* taking action. Indeed, it may well be that a sophisticated addiction to *talking about* taking action in fact inhibits our essential capacity to transform words and numbers into deeds. The more we spend on formal business education the more we multiply symbols and the longer action may be delayed.'

Secondly, this industrial programme shows great diversity in the designs of its score of projects. Some managers worked full time for about seven months on problems outside of GEC altogether; others left their own company to work out the problems of other GEC companies; some looked at problems elsewhere in their own company, others at particular developments that impinged upon their everyday job; a few even took that very job itself as their project. This last must pose the ultimate question: 'How can we all learn to see our normal work as a learning opportunity?' This at least is clear: the stresses set up within the hospitals of London demand that, whatever final benefits may flow from action learning (even if Part Three suggests they may be worth seeking), we must understand more clearly than we now do the relations between superior and subordinate. When the understrapper, by his personal involvement in the field studies, begins to descry and to advocate such remedies as may be called for, he has already created for himself a power that, to his boss, may be at best ambiguous and at worst abhorrent. It is, in general, difficult to sustain such a relationship; authoritarian regimes (as Janet Craig remarks on page 152) do not like power to be generated from below. But GEC, unlike the National Health Service, is not only a most flexible organization but one in which senior management cannot rely upon custom, practice or tradition; it must solve its problems as soon as it can, and has no time for discussions about status or precedence. Thus, although its bosses may wince at the first onslaughts of their evangelizing juveniles, they are sufficiently concerned for the performance of their undertakings not to dismiss suggestions simply because they are new. Indeed, as in many engineering companies, so overriding is the need in 1976 for simple economic survival that the action proposals of the manager-participants remaining in their own GEC jobs have thrown new light on the vertical communications of industrial hierarchies. 'Integrity of information' has become the slogan of fervent and interested debate.

The India Project

The Bureau of Public Enterprise, controlled by the Ministry of Finance of the Government of India, monitors over 100 nationalized industries and is aware of its problems of managerial development. It therefore resolved to set up, in 1975, a pioneer programme in action learning based on the temporary exchange between different industries of senior managers likely within three years to become directors of their own enterprises. As soon as possible after the start of this programme, whose participants will be designated as Jawaharlal Nehru fellows, its opportunities will be thrown open to the senior branches of the Civil Service and to certain enterprises controlled by the several states and larger municipalities; three or four national academic institutions of university rank will organize the project sets in which the essential exchanges of experience will occur. It is anticipated that the hospital services of India will be deeply involved in the programme, and that they will gain much, not only from Indian industry and from other Indian hospitals, but also from some of the ideas thrown up by the projects described at length in this book.

The Panchayat Project

The most interesting, certainly the most unexpected, consequence of the HIC Project, however, is a proposal, among the economic development plans of the Government of Bihar, to raise the quality of life in the villages of that vast region. What is called for is not only the better use of the resources of the soil, but also an improvement in the national administrative infrastructure to integrate more effectively the village and the factory; if the industrial masses of India need more food, so do the villagers, in order to grow it, need more of what industry can appropriately manufacture. The Bihar programme therefore proposes that the villages must first determine their own needs. To identify these, a sample of, say, 20 villages differing widely in natural endowment will, through their panchayats (village councils), help each other to identify both their needs and the resources necessary to meeting them. (Similar exchanges were designed into the HIC Project, but it was not before the end of the programme that their importance as a learning vehicle was grasped.) Needs might be found in many departments of village life, from education or health care to irrigation or the storage of crops, from the improvement of roads to the supply of fertilizers; an essential product of their identification will be to establish priorities in trying to fulfil them. Another output from these exchanges might be a clearer list of potential resources, such as improved marketing of produce leading to a higher village income. (Subsequent visits showed that the panchayats of two villages close to Delhi were at once attracted by the possibilities of discussing their own needs with the panchayats of other regions of the country.)

178

As the needs and resources of the 20 or so villages become clear from this first stage of the action learning programme, those items demanding interaction outside the village culture will be identified as clearly as possible: they are of two kinds, services or supplies to be brought into the villages from outside, and products or raw materials to be sold to the outside by the villages.

Six months after the start of the activities of the 20-village consortium, therefore, its findings will be fed into a consortium of about 20 appropriate organizations able either to supply the villages' needs (small industries, local public administrations) or to purchase their products (local tradesmen, commercial cooperatives). These organizations will, exactly like the 20 villages, work together on action learning lines, in order to identify among themselves how more effectively to service the villages (in both directions); their projects will be based upon the identified priorities of the villages themselves. This commercial, industrial and administrative consortium of the second rank will then pass its own ranked needs and resources upwards to a third-order consortium of about the same number of members in the field of heavy industry, wholesale commerce and regional administration. This third-order consortium will, in its turn and after an appropriate lead time, refer its needs and resources to a national consortium, largely of government organizations concerned with the public and economic infrastructure of the country.

Conclusion

This catalogue of references to eight major action learning projects suggests that we may approach our needs for managerial development and for institutional revival by a simple inversion of strategy. Instead of teaching (or attempting to teach) a canonical syllabus of technical theorems first and seeking its application to problems of management practice thereafter (the sequence determined by a culture of booklearning), we find out, by attacking the practical problems first, what we need to learn in order to overcome them. Some of these deficiencies, we note, may be outside our canonical syllabus, and some of our canonical syllabus may have no significant relation to our practical problems. In either event, we could change the items in our syllabus. But instead of continuously tinkering with what should be in the syllabus and what should be relegated to the index, why not start by attacking each practical problem itself and continue by consulting whatever entries in the whole encyclopaedia of knowledge it seems necessary to consult? We learn in the act of solving our problems and not in advance of knowing what those problems are.

The following paragraphs appeared in the *Bulletin of the European Foundation for Management Development* for May 1975:

'It could be argued that:
(a) Improvements in postgraduate education have now reached some kind of plateau and teaching methods and course content have for the most part not made the radical changes that were discussed so hopefully some years ago.

(b) Considerable initiatives are needed if research into the processes of management and the related specialisms is to improve in quality to the point where it can make a more direct contribution to understanding social and organisational activity. We have still further to go if we are to look for any dependable assistance with prescription.

(c) Management studies are susceptible to the same kind of criticism as has been levelled at the more quantitative management sciences, namely that they have too easily accepted current or outdated norms and views as bases for both teaching and research.

(d) The subject area is still defined in a way that discourages effective participation from a trade union point of view.

(e) Relatively little progress has been made with questions of utilization and applicability, notwithstanding the real efforts on the part of both educational institutions and industry.'

The essence of these chilling observations is that academic knowledge tells us increasingly little about management practice. Might we not try giving our first attention to that practice? We could then find out what we ought to know. As Abraham Lincoln remarked, the order of things may be important, and a horse chestnut is not just the same as a chestnut horse.

References

1. Mailick, S. (ed.), *The Making of a Manager: A World View*, pp. 132–5. Anchor Press/Doubleday, New York, 1974.
2. Musschoot, F., *Action Learning in Small Enterprises*, ALP Publications, Southport, Lancs.
3. Revans, R. W., *Studies in Factory Communications*, ALP Publications, Southport, Lancs.
4. Ashmawy, S., and R. W. Revans, *The Nile Project*, ALP Publications, Southport, Lancs.
5. Baquer, A., and R. W. Revans, *But Surely That is Their Job?*, ALP Publications, Southport, Lancs.
6. Drake, A. W., et al., *The Analysis of Public Systems*, MIT Press, 1972.
7. *Management Today*, p. 62, May 1975.

PART FIVE

Development in the health services—
action studies, participation, and involvement

by Dr Nelson F. Coghill

15. Development in the health services—action studies, participation, and involvement

Man, so quick to develop technology to apply the fruits of science, not least in medicine, is slow to understand the consequential social effects. Development in the Health Service is an index not only of social assimilation of technology, but also of ability to modify the working environment and to improve patient care.

On the basis that failure to recognize institutional unhappiness is to ensure that its causes go unmodified, we may look critically at activities in the hospital as a workplace. Experience indicates that people are capable of noticing that their working environment is less than satisfactory, of understanding how and why this is so, and of suggesting practical ways to improve it.

Doctors are enjoined to 'treat the whole patient'. Let us look at the hospital, the 'institution'—that abstraction that comprises staff and patients—also in the round and try to see where it is going, how it is working, what are its values and achievements, where are the defective relationships, what are the causes of its malfunctioning. The work in Lancashire hospitals described in this book and the subsequent studies of the HIC Project[1,2] indicate that these are the kinds of question to which managers should now be seeking answers. How better than to start by examining communication systems?[3]

Communication

Availability of information about their work is for most people a cardinal factor in the satisfaction they derive from it.[4] Changes in organization, designed to facilitate communication, may prove useful. But management may be too exclusively concerned with structure: if parts of the organization are rearranged, it is suggested, all will be well. Although human institutions have been shown at Brunel University to be almost invariably organized in hierarchies,[5,6,7] human attitudes and relationships cannot be changed or improved solely by altering the managerial structure and the mechanics of communication. In short, communication means more than the simple passing of information by mechanical means.

We do not know much of what actually happens when someone attempts to manage, but actions carry messages and emphasis on superior–subordinate relationships conveys the implication of inferiority to a very large number of people. Attention to the physiology and pathology of institutional behaviour will help people to work more effectively and productively. In all work, aims and interests are shared by all parties concerned in it. Instead of the cooperative activity that should characterize human enterprise, our commerce and services are run with workers, managers and consumers in watertight compartments, separated and polarized. The organization of work is thus bedevilled by the constant need to reconcile opposing interests; confrontation between different sides of industry is not conducive to the give and take so basic to agreement.

To be effective, communication must be a two-way process between individuals and groups, laterally and vertically. In a communication system there will always be two or more parties. All must listen as well as speak; all must be influenced. That is to say a communication system is properly a learning system. Attitudes may have to change for learning to occur, and for subsequent action to result. In a traditionally authoritarian hierarchical organization, a description fitting most hospitals, authority is an effective quencher of ideas and of upward communication. The young nurse who starts her training with the adjuration that she should not speak directly to a consultant, but only communicate with her ward sister, is being told that the consultant is not interested in any observations she may wish to make. If her ability to observe and communicate is inhibited, the quality of her training will be impaired, the consultant will lose the fresh insights of a student idealistically motivated to learn, and the young nurse will receive a lesson in how to become authoritarian. (Nurses receive little training in the scientific method and develop too much deference for the doctor. As a result, when qualified, even as sisters, they do not always feel able to communicate fully with the consultant. But this is changing.) If 'management' wants to persuade people who actually do the work (from student nurses, cleaners and porters to ward sisters, administrators and doctors), to work more effectively it should listen to what they have to say and be prepared to act upon it.

Control

Whatever the organization, whether it is run as a private enterprise, as an industry or service in public ownership, or as a workers' cooperative, the question of control is crucial. In most sorts of enterprise, strategic decisions have to be made about the running of the concern; their purpose should be clear and designed for acceptable social ends: where there is no will there is no progress. But the methods used to reach decisions, and the decisions themselves, must be acceptable to those whose duty it is to carry them out. Otherwise several possibilities arise: the decisions may be wrong; workers may decline to implement them, or to do so fully; or workers may, as a symptom of alienation, simply do the work badly, or leave.

The decision-making process is integral. With meaningful communications, and people at all levels accepting that they are in a constant learning environment, it is more likely that decisions will be made, correctly made, and properly implemented. Nevertheless, to achieve these ideal conditions of work implies the need for considerable changes in organizational methods at present in use in most human enterprises, and certainly in hospitals. The concept of control is one of the keys to understanding how people may work together more effectively. At present it has somewhat different meanings at different levels. Top management may see it as the way to ensure that its decisions are correctly implemented. Middle management may conceive it, perhaps wistfully, in terms of the power it ought to have to influence those above who are making policy decisions. To most at shopfloor level, control is a utopian idea that they seldom think of. Yet the shopfloor is able to spike management's guns by the negative, socially hurtful, actions of striking or sabotage. When a concern is threatened with closure and experiences a 'sit-in', this is a conscious effort by the workers to control their work-situation.

People's desire for control over their working lives is understandable for it offers them a sense of security and of identity. At work, confrontation between employer and employed would be ameliorated if means could be found to bring everyone into the design and control of their own lives. The conflicts in industry and services, which we constantly experience, offer evidence in plenty of the need for a wider acceptance of this truth. Nevertheless one man's control is another's constraint. So the questions are: How much control? To what extent? By whom, of whom? Can these implied incompatibilities be reconciled?

Learning

The studies described in this book, the experiences of later work stemming from the HIC Project,[8,9] Revans' work in Belgium,[4,10] and his studies of the care of the mentally handicapped,[11,12] suggest an answer to our conundrum; a solution, moreover, which not only appears to offer greater satisfaction to men and women at their work, but also one which may render the work more effective.

We have mentioned the process of learning in the work situation, what has been termed 'action learning'. If, in her encounter with the serpent, Eve had known more about serpents she might have been more circumspect. She found herself in a thoroughly authoritarian hierarchical institution (the Garden of Eden) (*Genesis*, ch. 2, vs. 15–17) in which, ironically enough, she and Adam were forbidden to eat the fruit of the Tree of Knowledge (we may absolve the Deity: the picture of Him is merely that in the minds of the people of the time); and of course the serpent also was not concerned to make the encounter a truly learning one: he wished only to persuade Eve to a course of action for his own ends. Man must order his affairs in less manipulative ways. I am concerned merely to stress the value of action learning, and more particularly, that it is a process that all may engage in, including the worker—whoever he or she may be—on the shopfloor, wherever or whatever that is.

There is little tradition for workers to offer their thoughts on how the shopfloor might be run, and so it is understandable that workers usually don't bother to have such thoughts. There are some essential prerequisites for action learning. The management structure must encourage and facilitate it. The workplace must be actively organized to produce the conditions for it to occur. To all these necessary changes there is built-in resistance from people who staff the authoritarian institution and have usually been trained in it. Authoritarianism is catching, as anyone may observe in a hospital where young doctors and recently qualified nurses display signs of it (Thus the resident doctor, who on failing to receive his early morning cup of tea, rang the fire alarm.) Inexperienced nurses and doctors naturally react with anxiety to situations fraught with uncertainty that are run of the mill in hospital life. It may sometimes be appropriate to react by issuing orders; but there are many circumstances when it would be more helpful for all involved patiently to explore the intricacies of the individual or group experience and extract from it the lessons without which there can be no personal or institutional development.

The concept of 'arena management' introduced by T. D. Hunter,[13, 14] may also help to improve worker effectiveness. Here the workplace is arranged as a 'locale', with people interrelating horizontally, rather than vertically. In different situations, and in the same one at different times, different people may become the focal point of the work. This does not mean that up–down and down–up relationships are not also required, particularly in planning institutional strategy. But it is with the work at shopfloor level that arena management offers advantages. It leads to the formation of a team, the supportive value of which is most evident in anxiety-producing situations such as occur in the ward. Ideas and comments about their work are more acceptable to nurses and doctors if they come from members of the team they work in. Administrators of all kinds also have problems they cannot solve alone, are under pressures they may find intolerable, and like others may at times feel threatened. The members of an institution who have consciously organized their work on a team basis are better able to help individuals within it who are under strain, or feel threatened by change, than can be done in a non-supportive organization run on hierarchical lines with strict individual accountability.

Attitudes

People have feelings about what happens to them, and about others' actions which may seem to carry messages for them. Feelings engender attitudes, and attitudes govern actions, as was seen clearly in the studies in Lancashire hospitals described in this book. It is of such stuff that interpersonal and interdepartmental relationships are made.

We are beginning to see a fuller development of the relationships between the 'service' departments in a hospital and the clinicians. The service that exists between these professionals is not one way. Mutual collaboration over certain patients and kinds of work enlivens interest and helps in research. Joint weekly meetings to discuss clinical and other problems are admirable learning situations to which all parties contribute. Thus various professional workers in the hospital offer service to each other. The development of such communication may help recruitment to shortage specialities such as pathology, radiology, anaesthetics and geriatrics.

Some reorientation of attitudes is needed on the part of authority, workers

186

and public, The public must be informed about the things done for them, and done in their name. Workers are inhibited from passing information about their work and the places they work in. The public may not listen, and the media may not present the facts. Even professional workers are inhibited from talking about the difficulties of providing an adequate service: they are too busy; there is no tradition; it is 'rocking the boat'. Public criticism, by a doctor or nurse about their hospital's facilities, or by a teacher about her school, will, authority believes, infallibly cause the community to lose faith in the institution (the *Lancet* does not agree[15]). For others there is the Official Secrets Act. Private concerns are even more secretive. How much of all this is merely an attempt by authority to protect itself while pretending to protect the public? In the Health Service the new Community Health Councils, if they and the hospitals see themselves as allies rather than enemies, could provide a forum in which institutional shortcomings might be examined, and through which the public might indicate its feelings about health care priorities.

Hospitals are traditionally authoritarian institutions with a hierarchical structure. This was seen as oppressive by the student and pupil nurses in their discussion groups.[2] Continuing discussion with nurses in training suggests that this view is weakening, but only slowly. However, there are developments which illustrate the potential of professional initiative.

The hospital ward

The professional workplace that is a hospital ward offers an opportunity to put into practice the two concepts of action learning and arena management. Perceptive sisters and consultants have practised these methods for years without using the terms, without necessarily developing them fully, and without involving everyone. It is convenient for the ward sister to be the principal focal point. Many people come to the ward in the course of their work and may be welcomed into the arena, and become part of the team. Some will be less involved as to time and commitment than others. Relatives, and patients who are fit enough, also help on the ward and are part of the team. (A first-year nurse who was upset by the unexpected death of a patient was comforted more by some of the patients in the ward than by any of her colleagues. Thus the ward is a community, as well as a place for the exercise of teamwork. The patients are served, but they may also contribute.) It must be acknowledged that to practise a high standard of hospital medicine would be impossible without organizing the work in some measure on a team basis.

However, the pressure of clinical work, the efforts of the nurses to provide service to patients and doctors commensurate with their high standards of training in the face perhaps of unhelpful supporting departments, the uncertainties besetting the inexperienced doctor tired after long hours and curtailed sleep, may engender tensions which affect behaviour. Sister is preoccupied and abrupt, doctor is beset and thoughtless. Damaged relationships heal slowly or not at all. There is no sovereign preventive for these human predicaments, but the more a group of people with the common aim of caring for sick people weld themselves into a team by thought and consideration for each other and for the first objective of their work, the greater may be their awareness and perception of others' difficulties, and the easier it should be to withstand the uncertainties of hospital life.

My colleague Dr James Stewart and I, with our ward sisters, have been trying various devices to increase communication in the ward team. Following our study on patients' anxieties performed in the HIC Project we give to each patient a duplicated leaflet containing information about the ward, and about visiting, with the names and functions of *all* who work on the ward. Patients with certain disorders, for example coronary thrombosis, are given advice about their convalescence both verbally and in writing. They would remember only a small part of it without the written notes they take home with them; verbal advice about sexual matters could not well be given in the open ward anyway. There is more or less open visiting: it is a help for relatives to feed and exercise patients; and information from nurses and doctors, given on the spot, calms relatives and prevents small problems becoming large ones. Elucidation of social difficulties is easier for sisters, doctors and medical social workers when relatives are about in the daytime and this shortens patient stay. The morning briefing on the patients, given by the ward sisters for the nurses, may be attended by the domestic workers and orderlies who are regarded as part of the patient-care team. The sisters spend as much time as possible teaching the student and pupil nurses. On the consultants' ward rounds one or more nurses in training are usually present, and one of them may speak about the patient she is caring for and be involved in discussion of their problems, supported by sister. The object is to provide a stimulus for the student's clinical work, and to make her feel valued as a member of the team. There is a weekly ward case conference on the social problems of all patients, particularly in relation to their re-integration into the community. Sisters, doctors, physiotherapist, occupational therapist, medical social worker and district nurse take part. There is a weekly meeting over tea of all medical staff and sisters of the joint unit to discuss administrative matters. The close contact between senior and junior nurses, and between doctors and nurses, so basic for all the interaction we describe, is sometimes difficult to attain because of the 40-hour week and shortage of nursing staff.

'Counselling'

In the autumn of 1972 the Standing Conference for the Advancement of Counselling set up a working party to investigate the extent and nature of counselling facilities available to nurses. The working party decided that it should first ask nurses themselves what facilities were needed. I was privileged to attend a series of meetings arranged by Mrs Hazel Edwards at the King's Fund Centre, of senior and junior nurses from a wide variety of organizations. At the start there was confusion as to what 'counselling' was. There were many who saw it as mainly remedial. It came to be accepted that, apart from advice about

188

their training and career, nurses might need help on three counts. A very small number might be psychiatrically ill and would need to consult an appropriate doctor. A somewhat larger group might have difficulty in adjusting to a personal problem—family bereavement, home sickness, boy/girl friend unhappiness, personality clash at work—all of which might be partly due to immaturity: these could be helped by counselling, although this might be obtained by discussion with anyone who was interested and helpful, not necessarily from a counsellor specifically appointed for the task. Much the largest category concerned those in conflict with the institution. There could be circumstances when it might be absurd to 'counsel' such people merely to induce them to conform: this would not alter the cause of the trouble and might leave an unredressed grievance. The group of nurses saw that it might sometimes be the institution that most needed 'counselling' and further that it might be the nurse, even the student nurse, who, in the thick of the experience, would be the appropriate person to do it.

This group of nurses grasped that the basis of 'counselling' was learning: learning about the problems of other people both as individuals and in a group (the 'institution'); and learning not least about the self. Several of the student nurses in the group, with support from their seniors and of the group, spontaneously initiated studies of various kinds: one into reasons why her peers were leaving; one into an attempt to start ward discussion groups; a third into the effect of ward 'atmosphere' on the learner. The results of these studies were presented to a final full meeting of all the members of the group. Simple research was here a valuable method of institutional self-learning.

That such ideas can be formulated and discussed by a group of nurses of mixed rank indicates clearly the capacity of professional people to understand the problems of their working lives when they are given an unfettered opportunity to discuss them together in a non-threatening supportive environment. But what of the practical application of these ideas? Implementation is ever the most troublesome stage of innovation. For centuries the ordinary worker on the shopfloor and the student (and the nurse in training is both) have been conditioned to accept their state without argument. Students may rebel, but student nurses merely leave: the wastage rate among student nurses is higher than that among any other type of student. Those in authority readily feel threatened at talk of change and the traditional attitudes of senior nursing staff set the stage for continuation of the *status quo*. We can hope to change these attitudes only by a deliberately supportive system of teamwork.

In my hospital we were concerned at the rate of student and pupil nurse wastage, at evidence of dissatisfaction and unhappiness among nurses in training, at authoritarian attitudes of senior nursing staff and at the number of unwanted pregnancies among nurses. After a year of discussions between senior nursing staff and others it was decided that, as general practitioner for 25 years to the nurses, I should talk to small groups of them at the start of their training about matters relating to their personal lives, to their status as students, and about relationships to their work, the patients, the hospital and the people they would work with. The nurses say they have appreciated these talks. The number of pregnancies has dwindled nearly to zero, but the effect on wastage has been much less certain. On the completion of their first year there has been a second meeting and on this occasion the nurses have made comments on a wide variety of their experiences at the hospital. The sisters have met in groups to be told about the approach to the nurses, and they have made many constructive comments. Thus the sisters were kept informed, they were offered an opportunity to contribute, and they were stimulated to think afresh about some of the many problems confronting a nurse in training. Nevertheless, without profound changes in staffs' attitudes a hospital remains an institution that discourages change. The same topics tend to be brought up by successive years of student nurses. It would be morale-depressing merely to continue indefinitely to listen to descriptions of the problems nurses encounter, without taking action. In most hospitals there is no ready made machinery for this. In an attempt to communicate across professional lines, hoping that action might follow, we set up an interdisciplinary group of nurses of all ranks, with some administrators and doctors. This unstructured 'cross-section' group meets monthly and has discussed problems common to more than one department, and items raised by junior nurses reflecting their attitudes to hospital life and experience. At another level we have started an unstructured ward discussion group, meeting fortnightly at lunch-time. All who work on the ward are welcome to the meetings and a sandwich lunch is provided. Numerous topics of a wide variety have been discussed. These exercises may be seen as a part of the institution setting out to 'counsel' itself, but they are more than this.

Action learning as a management facility

In whatever way others define a manager, in the Health Service it is said 'All are managers now'. The statement implies that the people on the job should 'manage' their work situation—not only doctors but everyone who works in the Health Service (and if this is true, everyone who works anywhere). Action learning will usually take place within an overall plan involving decisions on strategy. Anyone who does a job is capable of observing that job's intricacies and constraints and how it might be done more easily or in a less degrading way, or even how it might be done quite differently and more effectively. Such a person is a 'manager' if he is allowed to bring his critical faculties to bear on his work, and his creative initiative to influence how it is done.[16]

No one can understand the difficulties resulting from breakdown of machinery, or of human relations, so well as those who meet them at the workface. The same people can learn, perhaps with help and encouragement at first, to find solutions to these problems. When it comes to implementation of the solutions, help from beyond the actual workplace may be required. It is at this point that defects of expertise and will of middle and higher management may be exposed. Action studies will then be needed to help the institution to learn.[4] Such studies must include examination of support systems for existing managers. Apart from hierarchical and authoritarian traditions with which we have to con-

190

tend, a block to acquisition of managerial functions by the shopfloor worker is the resistance to change exhibited by superior managers because of the threat they feel such changes pose to them. Most managers are vulnerable also to pressures from above and do not always get the support they need from their superiors. (In a seminar on 'support', members of a course for first-line managers were given, to discuss, accounts of episodes that had actually happened. Here is one of them, from a sister: 'I returned to my Casualty Department after supper break to find three youths had stripped my student nurse. Before I could get to the alarm bell they started assaulting me. I retaliated with the result that two of the youths were admitted for observation. The next morning I was sent for by my Senior Nursing Officer and severely reprimanded for being too aggressive.')

Doctors spend much time at professional meetings designed to examine critically their own and others' work, and to keep their professional knowledge up to date. Many conduct research. Why should not Health Authorities be given a statutory duty to conduct research into the design and operation of all branches of their activities? Local administrations are obliged to undertake financial audits and they are traditionally expected to encourage research in technical and clinical affairs. They should also be expected, indeed obliged, to investigate their own functioning, if need be in conjunction with other authorities and institutions. In this kind of enquiry it would be difficult not to involve at some stage all the people working in the service. Professional workers may provide initiative and support for studies of the working of their own institutions. Not least of the results might be the realization by employers that in some jobs work being performed was of a more responsible nature than was previously thought.[17]

We see our ward group ('horizontal') meetings as a study in management using action learning principles. Mr Stephen Cang of the Brunel Institute of Organisation and Social Studies attends the meetings and is helping to describe the nature and structure of the problems which emerge. Discussions of the results in conferences at Brunel and the King's Fund Centre have provided important insights both into the proper nature of management in hospitals, and also into consequences of its lack. It seems probable that when an interdisciplinary team delineates problematic or innovatory work situations it usually has the power, discretionary, sapiential or both, to resolve them. Examples are to be found on the ward in respect of internal matters, and at the District Medical Team. These are at the extremes of hospital management levels. What has emerged from the study so far is an appreciation of the power vacuum and the consequent lack of managerial potential, at middle levels. Here communication is almost entirely up and down professional hierarchies with few lateral links. Our cross-section meeting was a first attempt to get communication across professional lines. Currently we are examining this problem further, and are not alone in becoming aware of it.[18]

Institutional advance depends first on learning where change is needed, and secondly on devising machinery to secure it. We have mentioned ways of obtaining information from the grass roots. We wonder if any 'management' will be realistic or effective not only in the devising of administrative machinery but also in the working of it, that does not embrace the active cooperation of all relevant workers irrespective of departmental or professional boundaries. A good example of action learning was a study in a mental hospital whose staff were concerned at the effects of visiting on patients and staff.[19] Wishing to understand better what these effects were and how they might be controlled or modified the hospital set up a well-organized interdisciplinary action study and quickly obtained some rather unexpected but useful results, helpful for both patients and staff.

Action learning can be applied in many ways.[2] We have been introduced to a form of 'worksheet' in use experimentally at Northwick Park Hospital. This is designed to record data about factors thought to govern length of patient stay and at the same time to help the nursing staff in their ward work: it is they who have been mainly concerned with its development, though some doctors have been involved. During the process of modifying the worksheets, nurses of all grades have gazed with more understanding at their work and have gained new insights into parts of it previously taken for granted.

From the same hospital we have learned of interdisciplinary 'user groups', set up to examine specific hospital activities and functions and consisting of people concerned with them. They may be *ad hoc* or on-going. In this way the effectiveness of a department or service within the hospital may be continuously monitored and feedback provided for its modification and improvement. Worksheets and user groups are examples of turning experience in the work place into learning situations, making use of simple cybernetic feedback loop systems. The process of learning results in improved working arrangements.

The role of trades unions in developing industrial democracy needs exploring. They have been concerned with rates of pay and safety conditions and by tradition tend to adopt a polarized stance of confrontation with management. However, they are now becoming more interested in the quality of life at work. To help them become involved in what to many shop stewards and union representatives may seem a new, uncertain and even threatening activity, management must be supportive in the working out and application of shopfloor participation and involvement. There is potential in middle management. At my hospital, at meetings of Heads of Departments, the principle of worker involvement has been received enthusiastically. The more difficult task of implementation has now to be tackled.

Much of this is not new. Doctors are concerned with research and the results of their work. Many people do work together in hospitals in a harmonious servicing manner; they are responsive; they will offer service when the need is plain and their work is valued. Studies indicate that many consultants are prepared to spend thought and time on improving the working of their own departments and hospitals even though this might entail examining their own actions.[2,8,9]

What is new is the increasing appreciation of the need for a greater scale and speed of social development in medical institutions.[20] It may seem elementary to have emphasized so many of these simple things, but it has to be admitted that many hospitals are anxious and sometimes unhappy places for patients and staff. We must appreciate the basic part that communications, attitudes, and participative management play in the development of harmonious and productive arrangements for work.

We have reached a stage in hospital practice when nurses and doctors are able to keep their professional knowledge and its practical application up to date, in spite of rapid advances in medical technology. Now we have to accelerate learning processes for social development. I think we shall see that the second is a necessary adjunct to the first.

References

1. Wieland, G. F., and H. Leigh (eds.), *Changing Hospitals. A Report on the Hospital Internal Communication Project*, Tavistock Publications, London, 1971.
2. Revans, R. W., (ed.), *Hospitals: Communication, Choice and Change. The Hospital Internal Communications Project seen from within*, Tavistock Publications, London, 1972.
3. Fletcher, C. M., *Communication in Medicine, The Rock Carling Fellowship 1972*, Nuffield Provincial Hospitals Trust, London, 1973.
4. Revans, R. W., *Developing Effective Managers. A New Approach to Business Education*, Longman, London, 1971.
5. Brown, W., and E. Jaques, *Glacier Project Papers*, Heinemann, London, 1965.
6. Kogan, M., S. Cang, M. Dixon, and H. Tolliday, *Working Relationship within the British Hospital Service*, Bookstall Publications, London, 1971.
7. Rowbottom, R. W., 'Emerging patterns of hospital organization', *British Hospital Journal and Social Services Review*, May, 1971.
8. Coghill, N. F., R. W. Revans, F. M. Ulyatt, and K. W. Ulyatt, 'A study of consultants', *Lancet*, **2**, 305–8, 1970.
9. Anderson, J. A. D., N. F. Coghill, G. S. A. Knowles, R. M. Pinder, R. W. Revans, and F. M. Ulyatt, 'Consultants' role in hospital management', *Medical Officer*, **125**, 73–7, 1971.
10. Revans, R. W., *The Theory of Practice in Management*, Macdonald, London, 1966.
11. Revans, R. W., and A. Baquer, *I Thought They were Supposed to be Doing That*, Comparative Study of the Coordination of Services for the Mentally Handicapped in Seven Local Authorities, June 1969 to September 1972, THC 72/735, King's Fund Centre, London, 1972.
12. Cortazzi, D., and A. Baquer, *Action Learning*, THC 72/736, King Edward's Hospital Fund, London, 1972.

13. Hunter, T. D., in H. Freeman and J. Farndale (eds.), *New Aspects of the Mental Health Services*, p. 73, Pergamon Press, Oxford, 1967.
14. Hunter, T. D., 'Self-run hospitals', *New Society*, **10**, 356, 1967.
15. *Lancet*, **1**, 190, 1972.
16. Coghill, N. F., 'Management in health services', *Lancet*, **1**, 1063, 1974.
17. Gooch, J. H., R. A. F. Harcourt, J. F. R. Ibbetson, and D. A. Whitmore, 'The hospital consultant's secretary', *British Medical Journal*, **3**, 456, 1972.
18. Kirk, C., and A. E. Bennett, 'Management and advice at the grass roots', *Lancet*, **1**, 1180, 1975.
19. Davis, D. E., 'Visiting groups: blessing or curse?', *Nursing Times Occasional Paper*, **71**, 5, 1975.
20. Coghill, N. F., 'Change and growth in hospitals', *Lancet*, **2**, 1058, 1969.

Index

Communication—*contd.*
    nature and need, 5, 28, 30–31, 39–40, 52, 77, 118, 128, 129, 131, 191
    nursing staff, 184
    (*see also* Interpersonal relations)
Community health councils, 187
Community health staff, 155
Computers, use:
    HIC, London Hospital, 138, 142
    HIC, North Middlesex Hospital, 146
Conditions of service, nursing staff, 17
Conferences:
    inter-disciplinary, in hospitals, 118
    HIC, Lewisham Hospital, 131–3
    senior staff, 144
    on wards, 58–9, 188
Conflict in hospitals, 154, 189
Consortia:
    Belgium, 172–4
    Bihari villages, 178–9
Constraints, financial, on surveys, 147, 148
Consultants, and the learning relationship, 71–2
    relationships with general practitioners, 68, 69
    relationships with nursing staff, 6, 57, 58, 61, 101–3, 188
    relationships with ward sisters, 57, 58, 61
    variations between, in patient stay, 21
Consultative committees, 76
Control, problem, in health services, 184–5
Convalescent homes, use by hospitals, 19–20, 23
Conversations on wards, 30–31
    (*see also* Communication)
Coordination of services for the mentally handicapped, 150–2, 175–6
Coronary thrombosis, advice for patients, 188
Counselling, 188–90
Courses, HIC project, 127, 129–30, 136
Craig, Janet, 164, 176, 177

Dallas, Southern Methodist University, 125, 174
Death rates (*see* Mortality rates)
Decision making process, in hospitals, 184–5
Delegation, need for, 172
Delhi, 178
Department of Community Medicine, 121
Department of Health and Social Security, 117
Dewey, John, ix
Diagnostic groups (*see* Patients)
Dining rooms (*see* Canteens)
Discharge of patients (*see* Patients: discharge)
Dissemination of information (*see* Communication)
District medical teams, 191
Doctors (*see* Consultants; General practitioners)

Domestic staff, wastage, 15–18
Domiciliary health services and length of hospital stay, 155
Drug administration, 141

Eastern Nigerian project, 169–70, 173, 175
Ecôle de Commerce, Brussels, 174
Economies, through shorter patient stay, 164
Education (*see* Nursing education)
Edwards, Hazel, 188
Egypt, 174–5
Emergency admissions project, 136, 137–40, 141
Enfield College of Technology, 146
Enugu, 170, 171
Essential change, concept, 173
Establishment ratios, 65–6
European Foundation for Management Development, 179–80
Evaluation, of Hospitals Internal Communications Project, 121, 159–65

Fairey, M. J., 135–42
Fatigue, of nurses, 37, 38
Feedback loop, information flow, 79
Fellows:
    Inter-University project, 173
    India project, 178
Finance, of HIC, 120–21, 127
    savings by shortening patient stay, 164
Financial constraints on surveys, 147, 148
Food; nurses' attitude towards, 36
Food supply, Bihar, 178–9
Freud, Sigmund, 82

GEC (*see* General Electric Company)
Garden of Eden, 185
Gastrectomy patients, hospital stay, 19–25
General Electric Company (GEC) programme, 176–8
General Nursing Council, 154
General Practitioner, Hospitals and Community, 155
    relationship with hospital medical staff, 68, 69
Good patients, 72
Group dynamics, 77
Guy's Medical School, 121, 122

HIC project (*see* Hospitals Internal Communications project)
Hawthorne effect, 164
Health services:
    action learning in, 190–93
    attitudes, 186–7
    communication, 183–4
    control in, 184–5
    counselling, 188–90
    developments since HIC, 183–94
Hernia repair patients, hospital stay, 19–25

199